Deafness

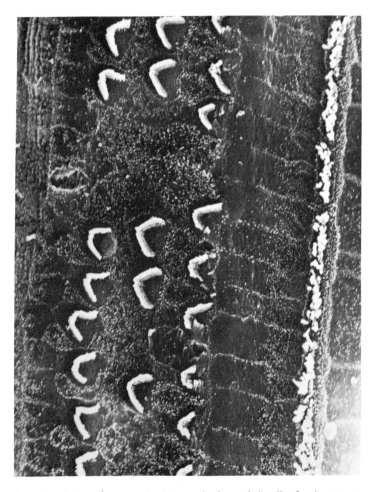

Scanning Electron Microscopic photograph of some hair cells of an inner ear damaged by exposure to noise. In a normal ear, the pattern of the hairs has a beautiful symmetry; in the cells damaged by noise, the hairs are distorted or absent. *(This photograph is reproduced by courtesy of Professor Hans Engström, of Uppsala University in Sweden.)*

DEAFNESS

John Ballantyne F.R.C.S., Hon. F.R.C.S. (I)

*Consultant Ear, Nose and Throat Surgeon to the Royal Free
Hospital and King Edward VII Hospital for Officers, London;
Honorary Civilian Consultant in Otolaryngology to the Army;
late Consultant Ear, Nose and Throat Surgeon to the Royal
Northern Hospital, London; late Assistant Director, Audiology
Unit Royal National Throat, Nose and Ear Hospital, London;
late Consultant Otologist, London County Council.*

THIRD EDITION

CHURCHILL LIVINGSTONE
EDINBURGH LONDON AND NEW YORK 1977

CHURCHILL LIVINGSTONE
Medical Division of Longman Group Limited

Distributed in the United States of America by Longman
Inc., 19 West 44th Street, New York, N.Y. 10036 and by
associated companies, branches and representatives
throughout the world.

First Edition   1960
  Reprinted   1961
Second Edition   1970
Third Edition   1977

ISBN 0 443 01602 X

Library of Congress Cataloging in Publication Data

Ballantyne, John Chalmers.
  Deafness.

  Bibliography: p.
  Includes index.
  1. Deafness. I. Title. [DNLM: 1. Deafness.
WV270 Bl88d]
RF290.B17   1977   617.8   77-3104

Printed by New Art Printing Co., (Pte) Ltd. Singapore.

Preface to the Third Edition

The years that have elapsed since the last edition of this monograph
have witnessed a great upsurge of interest in the problems of the deaf
in the United Kingdom, not least through the efforts of Members of
Parliament, the Department of Health and Social Security and the
Medical Research Council.

In 1974 the Department of Health set up an Advisory Committee
on Services for Hearing Impaired People, of which I have had the
honour and privilege of being Chairman; and a little earlier, the
Medical Research Council appointed two Working Parties, one of
which has been considering research into the Epidemiology of Deafness, the other into Rehabilitation of the Deaf. More recently, after
the typescript of this new edition was submitted to the Publishers,
there came into being an Institute of Hearing Research, which will
co-ordinate research efforts into the many different aspects of hearing
and deafness.

There have been detailed improvements in the design and performance
of individual hearing aids, and a new series of behind-the-ear (BE)
aids is becoming gradually available through the National Health
Service to all who can benefit from them; radio aids are now being
used in a number of special schools and, for those with the most difficult forms of deafness, much work is being done on the development
and potential value of 'recoding' hearing aids.

Industrial noise-induced hearing-loss is now recognized as a
'prescribed' disease in a limited number of noisy industries, and there
is reason to hope that the categories of workers who may benefit from
compensation for such losses will be extended in the not-too-distant
future.

The principles and techniques of reconstructive surgery of the
middle ear are becoming increasingly well understood, and the various
procedures involved in the surgery of deafness have come within the
repertory of more and more otologists. Attention is now being turned
to the pioneering efforts of otologists and others in California to the
restoration of at least some acoustic cues, by the implanting of electrodes in the cochlea, to those who suffer from irreversible and
otherwise untreatable inner ear deafness.

There has been a steady development in our knowledge of almost
every aspect of deafness, with a major renaissance of electro-physio-
logical methods in the measurement of hearing. I have greatly extended

my treatment of objective tests of hearing, and in this I have received much help from Mr W.P.R. ('Bill') Gibson.

There has also been an enormous growth of interest in the rehabilitation of the deaf, and the British Broadcasting Corporation has already produced (and repeated) one excellent series of programmes under the title of 'I see what you mean'. The chapter on rehabilitation has been re-written and considerably extended; and there is an entirely new chapter on that most distressing of symptoms, tinnitus, so often an accompaniment to deafness.

Once again I am indebted to Miss Wendy Galbraith for reading the revised chapter on the deaf child and for many helpful suggestions. Mr R. Hawksley has again brought me up to date with some of the newer developments in hearing aids and he has been kind enough to lend me all the commercial instruments which appear in the photographs. Mr R. H. Pugsley has supplied me with the photograph of a small clinical audiometer, and the hearing protectors were lent to me by the Safety Products Division of Racal-Amplivox Communications Ltd. The Multitone Electric Company has now been absorbed into the organisation known as A & M Hearing Aids Ltd. and the Managing Director, Mr D. W. Greener, has permitted me to re-use a number of illustrations.

To all these friends I am extremely grateful.

Unfortunately, time and distance have prevented me on this occasion from seeking the help of Richard Bartle, who made all the drawings for the first two editions of this book, but I have been particularly fortunate in enlisting the skill of Mr Frank Price, the distinguished medical artist, who has executed all the new drawings.

Throughout my chairmanship of the Advisory Committee on Services for Hearing Impaired People I have received unfailing support from my colleagues at the Department of Health, from none more than Doctors John Brothwood and Annette Rawson and Mr Derek Nye, secretary of the committee; and throughout the production of this new edition I have been treated with the greatest courtesy by the staff of Churchill Livingstone.

The task of typing the revisions from my almost illegible manuscript has been undertaken by my Secretary, Miss Jennifer Cowe, with her customary efficiency and good humour.

Almost twenty years have now passed since my wife, Barbara, suggested that I should write the first edition of this monograph, and it is to her that I re-dedicate it with my undiminished affection.

London 1977   J.C.B.

Preface To The First Edition
Abbreviated

Why another book about deafness? Several have appeared, mainly from the other side of the Atlantic, since the end of the Second World War. So also have many articles, in the professional and lay press, on the many different facets of this 'most desperate of human calamities' —as Samuel Johnson called it. But no serious attempt has been made in this country to put between the covers of one book a really comprehensive, though not exhaustive, account of deafness, as it affects people of all ages, and in all its many aspects—medical, educational, psychological and sociological—to mention only the most important.

Whilst several books have been written for the lay reader, professional men and women working with and for the deaf have had to turn, in the main, to their own specialist journals; and it is not easy, for example, for the otologist to find out what he wants to know about the educational facilities for deaf children, nor for the teacher of the deaf to keep informed about the type of person, child or adult, who is likely to benefit one of the modern operations for the surgical relief of deafness. It is for them, primarily, that this monograph is written— for otologists, medical officers of the Public Health Services, family doctors and paediatricians, teachers of the deaf, educational psychologists, missioners for the deaf, audiology technicians, and health visitors; in short for those whose professional work may bring them into close contact with the deaf.

But it is hoped that the presentation, designed as it is for a wide variety of interests, will also commend it to some intelligent laymen— to the deaf and to parents of deaf children.

Why, then, a monograph? This is deafness as seen and heard through the eyes and ears of one single otologist—one, furthermore, who believes that he has had the unusual good fortune to be able to examine the problem from many different angles. Apart from the knowledge which comes to all in the practice of otology, it has been my privilege to work for five years as Assistant Director of the Audiology Unit in Gray's Inn Road, London—an appointment which brought me into close contact with teachers of the deaf, both in clinics and in special schools, with psychologists and audiology technicians, and with the extraordinarily fertile brain of the research otologist, Dr L. Fisch. I have also been honoured to serve on many committees and sub-committees of a wide variety of professional organizations—the National Institute for the Deaf, the National Deaf Children's Society, the British

Association of Otolaryngologists, the British Standards Institution, and the Society of Audiology Technicians. I have, moreover, had the good fortune to act as otological adviser to the Public Health Service of the London County Council and to the Tewin Water School for the Partially Deaf, in Hertfordshire.

These activities have brought me into close contact with workers in practically every branch of Audiology, but I believe that not the least of my qualifications for writing this book is the fact that I was brought up in a 'deaf' household, whose 'master' has lived for more than half of his four score years with the handicap of deafness.

This book could never have been written without liberal reference to the standard literature, especially to the otological textbooks edited by Scott-Brown, Watkyn-Thomas and Maxwell Ellis; to Hirsch's book on *The Measurement of Hearing*; and to the many writings of my old chief and very good friend, Mr R. Scott Stevenson.

Help and advice have been freely given by many of my friends and colleagues: by Wendy Galbraith, head teacher of the deaf at the Audiology Unit, who was kind enough to read and criticize the chapter on the Child Born Deaf; by Michael Reed, educational psychologist, who allowed me to describe his 'rhyming word-picture' test and advised me on many matters psychological; by Peter Tizard, paediatrician at the Hammersmith Postgraduate Hospital, who helped me with the general aspects of Haemolytic Disease of the Newborn; and by Dr Mary D. Sheridan, of the Ministry of Health, who let me use some of her excellent pictures on Hearing and Speech.

Dr P. Henderson, of the Ministry of Education, and Mr G. Lilburn, Secretary of the National Institute for the Deaf, were jointly responsible for providing me with the list of special schools and units for the deaf and partially deaf.

I believe it to be a virtue of this book that most, if not all, of the illustrations appear now for the first time. Mr B. Montague, of the Multitone Electric Company Ltd., was good enough to lend me two of the photographs; and Mr Edwin Stevens, of Amplivox Ltd., provided another two. With these few exceptions, I am particularly grateful to Mr D. J. Connolly, of the Department of Clinical Photography at the Institute of Laryngology and Otology, who has taken all the other photographs. Some instruments were lent to me by Mr G. Cathrall, of Down Brothers and Mayer and Phelps Ltd., the commercial hearing aids by Mr S. C. Ingram.

Last but by no means least, I must thank my wife, Barbara, for her encouragement. It was she who first suggested that I write this book—this at a time when I was about to finish my five years of 'apprenticeship' at the Audiology Unit. Many of my clinics there were attended by visitors—visitors from all walks of life— and many questions were asked. I have also received others in letters from colleagues from every corner of the globe, and some of them took several evenings to answer. 'Where can I buy those pitch pipes?' 'Would an operation be any good for Janet?' 'Will a hearing aid help me?' 'Why do you say that this is the sort of audiogram you expect to see in the spastic child? Where can I find all this?'

It is in answer to these, and many other, questions that this book has been written.

London, 1960   J. C. B.

Contents

Part 7   The Handicap of Deafness

Appendices

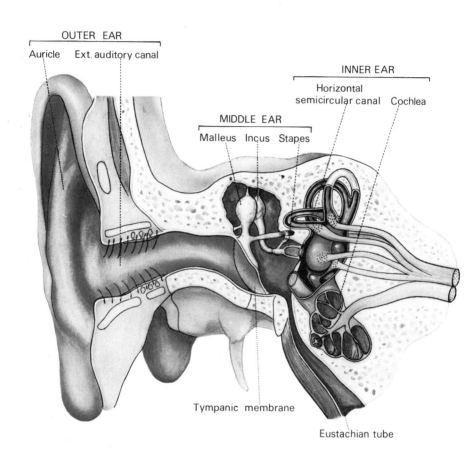

OUTER EAR

Auricle   Ext. auditory canal

INNER EAR

Horizontal
semicircular canal   Cochlea

MIDDLE EAR

Malleus   Incus   Stapes

Tympanic membrane

Eustachian tube

Fig. 1.1 Schematic diagram of the right ear.

1. The Incidence of Deafness

Since deafness is not a notifiable handicap in Britain, it is extremely difficult to arrive at a reliable estimate of its incidence. Further confusion is caused by the insistence of some authorities on drawing a distinction between 'total' deafness, 'profound' deafness, 'severe' deafness, 'partial' deafness of varying degress, and 'hardness-of-hearing'. There is no really satisfactory classification of the various degrees of deafness, and no two authorities will agree on where to draw the line between one degree and the next. It is only if we consider deafness as a whole—in all its degrees—that we can begin to reach something approaching an accurate idea of its incidence.

'It has been stated,' wrote Scott Stevenson, ' that there are six and a half million persons in England and Wales with some hearing defect in one ear or the other, but the extent of the problem of deafness in Great Britain has probably been more accurately gauged since the Social Survey Division of the Central Office of Information (Wilkins, 1949) carried out an investigation in 1947, primarily in order to provide an estimate of the number of Government hearing aids likely to be required under the National Health Service Act of July 1948. The report of the Social Survey was based on a set questionnaire concerning some 31 000 persons in England, Scotland and Wales *over the age of 16 years,* and interviews were carried out by trained field staff of the Social Survey who called upon the pre-selected subjects in their own homes.

This deafness survey was part of the 'Survey of Sickness' which is carried out monthly for the Registrar-General and the Ministry of Health, and names were drawn strictly at random from a geographically balanced and scattered, pre-selected number of maintenance registers. The data are supplied by informants about their hearing ability in response to standard promptings by investigators, so that the report is concerned mainly with the *complaints of deafness, whether real or imaginary,* and whatever their origin.

'The total number of deaf persons in the population of England Scotland and Wales was thus calculated to be 1 774 000, made up of 15 000 deaf mutes; 30 000 totally deaf; 70 000 deaf to all natural speech; and 1 659 000 hard-of-hearing persons, of whom 790 000 had difficulty in hearing normal direct speech without hearing aids, but could hear loudly spoken speech. The 70 000 'deaf to all natural speech' had difficulty in hearing loudly spoken speech, but could hear speech amplified by hearing aids or by other means.

Perhaps the greatest weakness of this survey was the subjective nature of its approach, and no further survey has been conducted on this scale since the Wilkins Report, although the National Health Service has now been in existence for almost 30 years.

Nevertheless, more up-to-date figures would suggest that this is no exaggeration and, in attempts to assess the number of people who will need the recently introduced behind-the-ear NHS hearing aid, it has been estimated that one-and-a-half to two million people in the United Kingdom suffer from some degree of hearing loss; and in a 'Report of a Departmental Enquiry into the Promotion of Research' published by Her Majesty's Stationery Office in 1973, Dr Annette Rawson suggested that probably some two million people of pensionable age alone must have an impairment of hearing. There are, however, no accurate figures for calculating the incidence of hearing loss in the population of employment age, and this must be a sizeable number, probably amounting to a further one million.

These figures give us little or no idea of the number of deaf and partially hearing children, in their school and pre-school years, but in a report to the National Deaf Children's Society, in 1958, J.B. Perry Robinson wrote as follows:

'There are approximately 6750 children in special schools and classes for the deaf or awaiting admission (5550 in England and Wales; 1000 in Scotland; 200 in Northern Ireland) and probably a further 500 in other institutions (hospitals, homes, schools for the educationally subnormal and spastic institutions), including about 40 deaf-blind. There may be as many as 3000 pupils in normal schools, including private Preparatory and Public Schools, who ought to have hearing aids or be in special classes.'

More recent *official* returns showed that the following numbers of children were being educated *in special schools:* in England and Wales (as at January 1967) 4797 pupils (3118 classified as 'deaf' and 1679 as 'partially deaf'); in Scotland (as at the same date) 726 pupils (414 'deaf' and 312 'partially deaf'); and in Northern Ireland (as at January 1968, one year later) 161 pupils (110 'deaf' and 51 'partially deaf')—a total of 5684 in the whole of the United Kingdom. And yet more recently a similar figure of children in special schools (4976) has been produced by the Secretary of State for Education.

Further analysis of the figures from England and Wales shows that 6 out of every 10 000 school-children have such severe impairment of hearing that they require special educational treatment in special schools; and two-thirds of these are educationally 'deaf', the remainder 'partially deaf', or (as they are called nowadays) 'partially hearing'. But these figures do *not* include those children who attend the 'Partially Hearing Units' (PHU's) attached to ordinary schools; and these amount to a further 2000 children in England and Wales, thus bringing up to a total of 8.5 per 10 000 the number of children of school age who require some form of special educational help.

In addition, there is a large number of children of pre-school age with hearing defects, and Perry Robinson estimated 'that there are altogether 15 000 to 20 000 pre-school-age children in the United Kingdom with serious defects and 30 000 to 40 000 who could do with some help'.

There must also be several thousands of children in ordinary schools, most of them with the lesser degrees of 'catarrhal' deafness, whose hearing fluctuates with the vagaries of the weather and the common cold; and the condition of 'glue' ear, although treatable and in most cases curable, is an extremely common condition which may produce a not inconsiderable handicap.

Of necessity, then, all such figures must inevitably be based more on intelligent calculations than on actual returns, but they do serve to emphasize that the handicap of deafness, at all ages, is much commoner than is often recognized; and attempts are now being made to arrive at more accurate estimates, by two working parties recently set up by the Medical Research Council.

2. The Structure of the Ear — Anatomy

This is a book about deafness, and its main purpose is to describe those clinical aspects of deafness which are the chief concern of the deaf themselves and of all those who work with and for the deaf. But we cannot describe the functional disorder which we call deafness without some understanding of the way in which the normal ear works; and we cannot describe its workings without a knowledge of its structure. This opening chapter will therefore be devoted to anatomy, for anatomy is the science of structure.

For descriptive purposes, the ear is divided into three parts — the outer ear, the middle ear and the inner ear.

The outer ear

The outer ear consists of the auricle (or pinna) and the external auditory canal (Fig. 1.1).

The *auricle* is the visible part of the ear and it has little function in man. It has a framework of cartilage, except in the soft lobule, and the folds and furrows of its skeleton are tightly clothed with skin.

The *external auditory canal* is a narrow, slightly tortuous passage which leads inwards from the 'base' of the auricle for a distance of about one inch in the adult. It is the only skin-lined cul-de-sac in the body, and the surface layers of keratin are shed in much the same way as the skin on other surfaces. Only in its outer part are there ceruminous glands (which secrete wax) and fine hairs. The deepest part of the canal is separated from the middle ear cavity by the tympanic membrane. Peter Alberti has shown that the skin on the outer surface of this membrane (see page 93) 'migrates' slowly from its central area towards the periphery, and ultimately out of the meatus. The overall rate of this migration is equivalent to that of the growth of a finger nail.

The middle ear cleft

The middle ear cleft (Fig. 2.1) appears as an outpouching from the primitive nasopharynx during the early months of embryonic development, and the cleft maintains this connection with the nasopharynx throughout life. Its first part is the *Eustachian tube*, which leads upwards, backwards and outwards from its lower opening in the nasopharynx to its upper opening into the middle ear cavity. The tube is almost one and a half inches long in the adult; normally closed at rest, it opens on yawning or swallowing. It is the route by which infections most commonly enter the middle ear cavity from the nose and, since the tube is relatively wider, shorter and more horizontal in children than in adults, it is not surprising that these infections occur much more commonly in infants and young children. The lower end of the tube is also said to contain some lymphoid tissue (the 'tubal tonsil') beneath the surface mucous membrane, but considerable doubt has been cast on the veracity of this long-accepted supposition. It *is* known, however, that there *is* some of this lymphoid tissue in very close proximity to the lower opening of the tube.

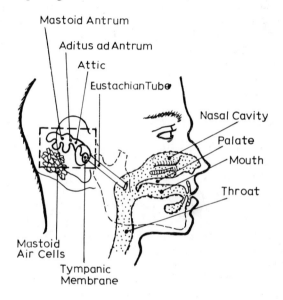

Fig. 2.1 The right middle ear cleft.

The *tympanic (middle ear) cavity* is a small cavity situated in the temporal bone on either side of the head. It has the form of a biconcave disc. From roof to floor, and from front to back, it measures only half an inch, and there is a distance of rather less than one-tenth of an inch between its outer and inner walls at the narrowest part of the cavity.

The greater part of the cavity is closed off from the external auditory canal by the *tympanic membrane* (or drumhead), but there is a smaller part, *the attic*, which lies above this level. The drumhead is set obliquely at the deep end of the external auditory canal and is concave outwards.

If we take away the tympanic membrane, and look in more detail at that part of the middle ear cleft which is contained in the square in Fig. 2.1, we can see the inner wall of the tympanic cavity, which is the bony party-wall between the middle ear and the inner ear (Fig. 2.2). Its most obvious feature is the *promontory*, which bulges outwards to narrow the cavity. There are two windows in this wall—an *oval window* above and behind the promontory, and a *round window* below and behind the promontory. The oval window looks more or less directly outwards into the cavity, but the opening of the round window is set obliquely and lies in a niche under cover of a small ridge of bone.

The main contents of the cavity are the three minute ossicles (Fig. 1.1), which take their names from the smithy's forge—the malleus (or hammer), the incus (or anvil) and the stapes (or stirrup). Their function is to transmit sound-waves from the surface of the drum-head to the oval window. The *malleus* has a head, a neck, a handle, and anterior and lateral processes. The handle is firmly attached to the tympanic

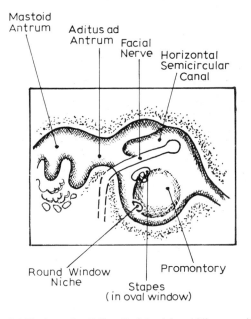

Fig. 2.2 The inner (medial) wall of the right middle ear cavity.

membrane, and the tendon of the *tensor tympani muscle* is inserted into its neck. The *incus* has a body (articulating with the head of the malleus) and a short process, both in the attic; it also has a long process which descends behind the handle of the malleus and parallel to it. This process bends inwards at its lower end, to form the lenticular process which articulates with the head of the stapes. The *stapes* has a head, a neck, anterior and posterior crura, and a footplate, the last named being held in the oval window by the annular ligament. Attached to the neck of the stapes is the tendon of the *stapedius muscle*, which takes it origin from a small bony nipple, the *pyramid*, in the posterior wall of the cavity.

The *aditus ad antrum*, as its name implies, is a narrow passage which leads backwards from the attic to the mastoid *antrum*. The antrum is a space which is found constantly in the posterior part of the temporal bone, and it lies at a depth of up to half an inch from the surface of the mastoid portion of the bone. The *mastoid process* is the rounded, bulbous process which lies behind the auricle, and 80 per cent of human mastoid processes are occupied by numerous *mastoid air-cells*, communicating with one another and with the antrum by many openings. These air-cells give a honeycombed appearance to the mastoid process when it is cut across, but in one person in five the cells are small or even absent. A mastoid process which is entirely devoid of air-cells is aptly described as the 'ivory mastoid'. The cause of these differences is not yet fully understood, but their significance will be discussed when we come to consider infections of the middle ear cleft.

The greater part of the middle ear cleft is contained within the petrous portion of the temporal bone—well named after Peter (a rock), for this is in fact the hardest bone in the body, with the one exception of dental enamel.

The entire cleft is lined by an uninterrupted sheet of mucous membrane, from the furthermost cells in the tip of the mastoid process to the lowermost part of the Eustachian tube, where it become continuous with the mucous membrane of the nose and throat, and indirectly, of the nasal sinuses. In health, the cleft contains only air.

Before passing on to a description of the inner ear, it should be emphasized that the only parts of the middle ear cleft which are

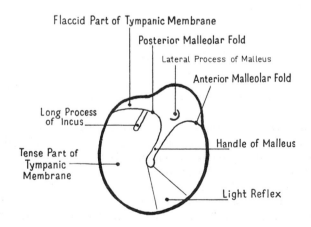

Fig. 2.3 Normal right tympanic membrane (drumhead).

accessible to visual inspection are the lower end of the Eustachian tube (which can be seen in the small post-nasal mirror introduced through the mouth) and the tympanic membrane (Fig. 2.3). So important are the changes which occur in the membrane, and so great is the information which can be obtained from its inspection, that a brief description of its main landmarks may not be out of place here.

It has already been said that the drumhead is set obliquely at the depths of the external auditory canal. Only one small segment of it is directly vertical to the examining eye, and the *light reflex* is formed by a reflection of the light cast by the examiner on this particular part of the drumhead. This is the most obvious landmark, and at its upper end lies the lowest part of the handle of the malleus, known as the *umbo*. The short *lateral process* of the malleus projects outwards from the upper end of the handle, and the *malleolar folds* pass forwards and backwards from this point. The long process of the incus may sometimes be seen behind the handle of the malleus, halfway between it and the posterior wall of the external canal.

The greater part of the membrane, below the malleolar folds, has three layers—an outer epithelial (or skin) layer; a tough middle fibrous layer; and an inner mucosal layer which is but a part of the membrane which lines the whole of the middle ear cavity. This tense part of the drumhead is known as the *pars tensa*. The middle fibrous layer is partially deficient in the small upper part of the membrane, above the malleolar folds, and it is known as the *pars flaccida*. This flaccid part (and possibly also the postero-superior portion of the tense part) is an area of relative weakness, compared with most of the tense part.

The inner ear

The inner ear is aptly known as the labyrinth—literally 'a structure of winding passages'. Functionally, it has two parts—in front, a hearing portion, the cochlea; behind, the utricle and semicircular canals, concerned with balance. Each of these two parts of the inner ear consists of a complex series of soft membranous tubes contained within a further complex series of bony cavities situated in the petrous part of the temporal bone.

The *cochlea* is so named from its resemblance to a snail-shell (Fig. 1.1). It has two and a half turns in the human. The oval and round windows are situated in the outer wall of its bony casing; and the promontory covers the first (or basal) turn of the cochlea.

Now let us look at the cochlea alone (Fig. 2.4, i) and split it along the line A—B. Open it up along this line of cleavage and enlarge it, and we shall begin to see some of the broad details of its internal structure (Fig. 2.4, ii). The soft membranous inner tube of the cochlea is the *scala media,* which contains the *endolymph* fluid, which has a high

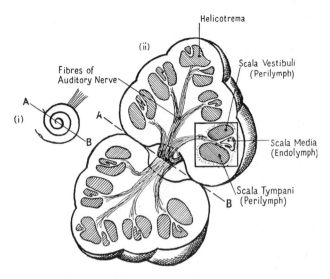

Fig. 2.4 The cochlea. (i) The 'snail shell'. (ii) Enlarged 'section' of the cochlea.

content of potassium and a low content of sodium, like the fluids within cells (intracellular fluids). Endolymph is the sole source of oxygen supply for the organ of hearing, which itself has no blood vessels. Separating this from the outer bony tube is the *perilymph* fluid which has a chemical composition generally similar to that of the fluids out-side cells (extra-cellular fluids), and it is continuous and identical with the cerebrospinal fluid, which surrounds and 'cushions' the brain and nerves. The upper chamber of perilymph is the *scala vestibuli,* which is closed by the footplate of the stapes and its annular ligament; the lower one is the *scala tympani,* which is closed by the *secondary tympanic membrane,* covering the round window. These two chambers of perilymph communicate with one another, at the apex of the cochlea, through the *helicotrema.*

If the windows were not closed, the perilymph could escape into the middle ear, and sound would not be transmitted into the cochlea.

Next, take that small part of the cochlea enclosed by the square in Fig. 2.4 and enlarge it even further (Fig. 2.5). Here, for the first time, we can see in some detail the minute sense organ of hearing itself. And we can see that the soft membranous inner tube of the cochlea (the *scala media*) is roughly triangular in shape, not circular. The base of the triangle is formed by the *basilar membrane,* which stretches across from the bony spiral lamina to the spiral ligament. Its outer wall contains the *vascular stria,* and it is from this fine network of capil-laries that the endolymph (so it is thought) is formed and partially re-absorbed. The third side of the triangle is formed by *Reissner's membrane*.

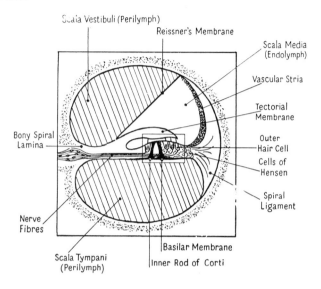

Fig. 2.5 Microscopic section of the cochlea (low power).

The *organ of Corti,* so named after the Italian Marquis, Alfonso Corti, is the sense organ of hearing and it sits upon the basilar membrane throughout the whole length of the membranous cochlea. It consists of a series of epithelial structures, of which the critical cells are the hair-cells. They are disposed in a single row of *inner hair-cells,* astride inner *rod of Corti,* and three or four rows of *outer hair-cells,* outside the outer rod of Corti. Between the inner and outer rods is the tunnel of Corti, which contains a third fluid which has been described and named by Hans Engström as the 'cortilymph'. In chemical composition it is much nearer to that of perilymph than of endolymph, but its exact origin and nature are not yet known. Minute 'hairs' project from the free surfaces of the hair-cells into the overlying, gelatinous *tectorial membrane* (Fig. 2.5). Supporting the outer hair-cells are the *cells of Hensen.*

But it would be wrong to think of the organ of Corti as a solid, motionless structure. Rather should we think of it as composed of a very large number of functionally independent units (four to five thousand of them in fact), each closely related to its neighbour but each capable (more or less) of independent movement. Some idea of this arrangement can be gained if we look at it under much higher magnification (Fig. 2.6). This drawing shows six of these units lined up in close proximity to one another and each connected with its neigh-

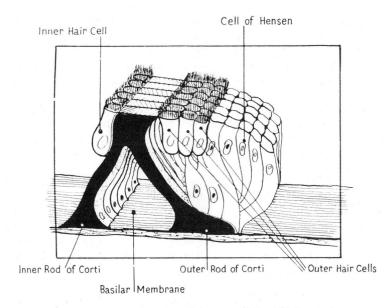

Inner Hair Cell

Cell of Hensen

Inner Rod of Corti

Outer Rod of Corti

Outer Hair Cells

Basilar Membrane

Fig. 2.6 Microscopic section of the organ of Corti (high power).
Six 'units' are shown.

bour by the continuity of the supporting basilar membrane, which
winds spirally up from base to apex for about one inch.

If each of the four or five thousand independent units of the organ
of Corti contains an average of four hair-cells, then the total number
of hair-cells in each ear will be between 16 000 and 20 000.

Afferent nerve fibres (Fig. 2.5) pass from the hair-cells, and they
number at least 30 000 on each side; but the relationship between the
hair-cells and these nerve fibres is far from simple, for each fibre
connects with several hair-cells, each hair-cell with several fibres. The
complexity of these arrangements has been beautifully demonstrated
by Hans Engström in his recent work with phase contrast and electron
microscopy.

After passing through the *spiral ganglia,* the thousands of afferent
nerve fibres become entwined together, like the strands of a rope, and
collectively they form the auditory nerve. This is the VIIIth cranial
nerve. It is in this nerve that the messages received by, and analysed
in, the ear are carried up to the brain, where their meaning is inter-
preted.

Apart from the 30 000 or more afferent fibres, there have also been
demonstrated some 500-odd efferent (or centrifugal) fibres which pass
to the hair-cells *from* the brain stem.

From the cochlea, afferent fibres of the *auditory nerve* (Fig. 2.7, A)
pass through the *internal auditory canal* to the cochlear nuclei in the

brain stem. Hence they pass upwards, through the brain stem and the brain substance, to the higher *auditory centres* in the temporal lobe of the brain. The efferent fibres appear to be linked, at the level of the brain stem, with the cochlear nuclei and to be controlled from cortical levels by descending fibres (Fig. 2.7, B). The significance of these centrifugal fibres is not yet fully understood.

Accompanying the nerve through the internal auditory canal is the *internal auditory artery,* the branches of which supply the labyrinth. These branches are end-arteries—arteries which make no connection with one another. In the absence of such anastomotic safety-valves, deafness may be caused by their occlusion.

The cochlea is so small that we have to resort to microscopical studies before we can describe it in detail; and after looking at a number of these pictures, it is not at all surprising that many of us will tend to have a grossly exaggerated conception of its size. To put this structure of winding passages in its proper perspective, we must try to retrace our steps and look once more at our first drawing of the labyrinth (Fig. 1.1).

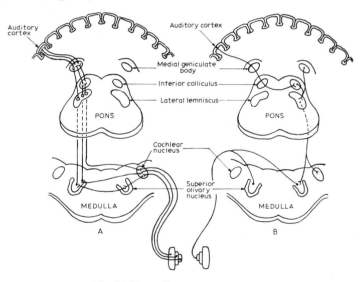

Fig. 2.7 The auditory nervous pathway.
A, Afferent fibres.   B, Efferent fibres.

It may not be quite so difficult, after looking at this drawing again, to convince ourselves that the whole of the cochlea from base to apex measures no more than one-fifth of one inch. Yet all of the thousands of hair-cells of the organ of Corti are contained within this incredibly small space, and every one of them is almost fully formed by the fourth month of embryonic life. It is, perhaps, only when we can learn to think of the cochlea in these terms that we begin to wonder how it is that so often it is perfect.

In a book about deafness, it is natural that much space should be given to a description of the cochlea, but a few words more must be said about the vestibular (or equilibrial) part of the labyrinth before we leave Anatomy. Particularly must mention be made of the *semicircular canals,* three on each side, which are set at right angles to one another and therefore represent the three planes of space (Fig. 1.1). As in the cochlea, each canal consists of a soft membranous tube within a hard bony tube. The most important of these canals, from the surgeon's point of view, is the horizontal semicircular canal which projects into the inner wall of the aditus ad antrum (Fig. 2.2).

Although it is customary to describe hearing and equilibration as two separate and distinct functions of the inner ear, it must be emphasized that the membranous inner tube of the cochlea and the membranous inner tubes of the semicircular canals all contain endolymph fluid; and that all parts of the membranous tubular system of the inner ear are in direct continuity, structurally and (to some extent) functionally. The importance of this fact and the relatively great importance to the surgeon of the horizontal canal will be understood when we come to describe labyrinthitis and the historical operation of fenestration.

3. What We Hear — Acoustics

Those of us who are fortunate enough to have normal hearing spend the greater part of our waking hours listening consciously or unconsciously to sounds. There may be the sounds of music or the noise of traffic, but above all, they are the sounds of human speech. All of them are complex sounds, which consist of various combinations of pure tones.

The physical characteristics of pure tones

Sound reaches the ear in the form of waves, which travel from their source at a speed of 760 miles per hour. Sound waves cause changes of pressure at the ear, and these changes alternate between increases of pressure (or compressions) and decreases of pressure (or rarefactions). One of these alternations (or double vibrations) of pressure is said to perform one cycle, but the human ear is unable to perceive sound waves *as sound* until the number of these alternations of pressure reaches twenty per second.

Frequency. Another way of expressing this is to say that the lowest tone which is audible to the human ear has a *frequency* of 20 cycles per second or hertz (Hz). As frequency increases we perceive a rise in *pitch*, and when it reaches 256 Hz, we hear a tone which has the same pitch as the note of middle C on the piano. If this frequency is doubled (to 512 Hz), the note produced will be one octave higher; if it is halved, the note will be one octave lower. The top note of the piano, top C, is four octaves above middle C and therefore has a frequency of 4096 Hz. As the frequency rises beyond this point, the note heard becomes shriller and shriller until, at 20 000 Hz, the sound is heard merely as a hiss. Finally, the sensation of sound disappears altogether at about 30 000 Hz.

If a note has only one single frequency (for example, 256 Hz) it is said to be a pure tone; and it produces what is know as a sinusoidal wave-form, or a sine wave (Fig. 3.1, A).

Intensity. In the same way as the sensation of pitch depends upon the frequency of the stimulating tone, so does the sensation of *loudness* depend upon its *intensity*. And just as the physicist measures frequency in cycles per second, so does he measure intensity in terms of decibels.

A tone which is only just audible is known as a *threshold* sound. The softest sound of human speech to which we normally listen is a whisper,

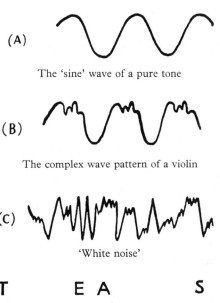

(A)

The 'sine' wave of a pure tone

(B)

The complex wave pattern of a violin

(C)

'White noise'

T   E A   S

(D)

Consonant   V o w e l   Consonant

The complex wave pattern of the spoken word 'Teas'

Fig. 3.1 Sound 'waves'.

and a whisper is about one thousand (1000) times more powerful than a threshold sound, at a distance of about three feet. A normal conversational voice at the same distance is about one million (1 000 000) times more powerful than a sound which is barely audible, whilst a loud shout is as much as one thousand million (1 000 000 000) times as powerful. The power of a sound which will produce discomfort in the ear is no less than one billion (1 000 000 000 000) times greater than the power of a sound which is just barely audible.

So enormous is this *range* of power with which the ear has to deal, that power ratios of tenfold have been introduced to express these levels. Named after the famous scientist Alexander Graham Bell, these units are known as bels. A threshold sound will be 0 bels. A whisper, as we have said above, is 1000 (10 × 10 × 10) times more powerful; alternatively, this can be written as 10^3, where the base (10) is raised to the power of 3. This power ratio of three is known as the exponent, and it is this exponent alone which is used when we measure power ratios in terms of bels. In the present example we can say, therefore, that a whisper is 3 bels louder than the threshold sound. Similarly a conversational voice will be 10^6 times (or 6 bels) louder, a loud shout will be 10^9 times (or 9 bels) louder, and discomfort will be felt when the sound is 10^{12} times or 12 bels) louder. *The number of bels will be the same as the number of noughts.*

In practice it is found that the bel is too large a unit, for we want to measure differences in hearing acuity with much greater accuracy. For clinical purposes therefore the bel is split up into ten smaller units known as *decibels,* and this is usually written as dB. Hence, to re-write once more the examples given above: a threshold sound will have a power of 0 dB; a whisper will be 30 dB louder; a conversational voice will be 60 dB louder; a loud shout will be 90 dB louder; and discomfort will be experienced when the stimulating tone is 120 dB louder than the threshold tone.

The decibel is a very convenient unit for clinical use, for it so happens that one decibel is (very roughly) equal to the least perceptible difference of loudness detectable by the human ear, in the frequencies concerned with our hearing of speech.

The measurement of hearing for pure tones – pure tone audiometry

The ability to hear pure tones can be measured on the audiometer. This consists essentially of four parts: an *oscillator,* which produces (electrically) tones of any desired frequency; a *frequency selector,* which delivers these tones either in fixed discrete frequencies (in octave or half-octave steps) or in sweep frequencies (delivering the complete band of frequencies from the lowest to the highest); an *attenuator,* which alters the intensity, usually in steps of 5 dB; and a *receiver,* which delivers the pure tones to the ear.

In its simplest form (Fig. 3.2), there are two main controls on the panel—one which allows the frequency of the tone to be altered (in octave or half-octave steps); and another which allows us to change its intensity (in 5dB steps). The sound is delivered to the ear by a headphone closely applied to the ear under test (air conduction); it is also possible to deliver the testing sounds to the mastoid process, whence they are transmitted through the bones of the skull to the cochlea (bone conduction). The frequencies range from 250 Hz to 8000 Hz in octave or half-octave steps (250, 500, 1000, 1500, 2000, 3000, 4000 6000, and 8000 Hz), and these figures are used, purely for simplicity, in preference to the less easily remembered figures of the musical scale (512, 1024, etc.). Each tone is presented separately, one ear at a time, and it is usual to start with an easily discerned tone, commonly of 1000 Hz. This is presented initially at a level of intensity which will be heard easily by the listener, so ensuring that he is certain of the exact pitch of the testing tone. When this has been established, the volume control is turned down gradually until the sound disappears. Finally the

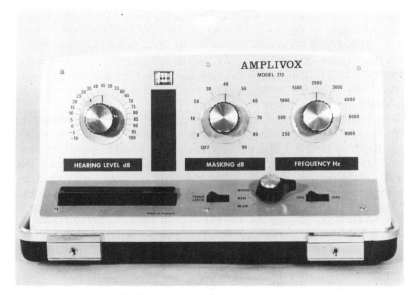

Fig. 3.2 A simple pure tone audiometer. (Amplivox portable.)

volume is turned up again once more until it is just barely audible. This gives us a measure of the threshold for hearing of the ear under test, and the same procedure is used for each of the frequencies mentioned until one ear has been completely tested. It is then repeated in the opposite ear and the result is plotted on a graph.

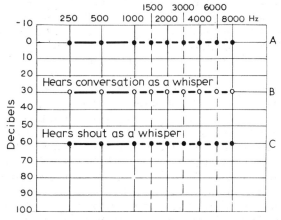

Fig. 3.3   The pure tone audiogram.

This audiograph or (more commonly) audiogram (Fig. 3.3), records the hearing loss in decibels for each separate frequency, and it will be seen that a person with normal hearing has a loss of 0 dB (A). It will be remembered that a whisper is 30 dB above the threshold level, a conversational voice 60 dB and a shout 90 dB above it. At a distance of 3 feet, the patient with a hearing loss of 30 dB (B) will therefore perceive a normal conversational voice as we, with normal hearing, hear a whisper; and he will perceive a shout as we hear the normal conversational voice. When the hearing loss is 60 dB (C), the patient will hear a shout only as a whisper.

In testing an adult, it is customary to ask him to indicate whether the testing tone is audible or inaudible simply by raising the hand, or saying 'Yes' or 'No'. Alternatively, he may be asked to press a button, to illuminate the testing panel, which can be seen by the examiner but not by the person under test. The technique employed with children differs in certain important respects and will be described later in the chapter on 'The Deaf Child; and the important subject of masking is discussed in the chapter on 'The Functional Examination of Hearing'.

The standardization of audiometers is a most important subject, the purpose of which is to ensure that tests of the threshold of hearing of an individual patient on different audiometers, each complying with a given standard, will give substantially the same results under comparable conditions, and that the results obtained will represent a true comparison between the threshold of hearing of the patient and the normal threshold of hearing.

It is therefore important to be able to determine a normal threshold of hearing and many attempts have been made to find the value of this threshold. By testing many hundreds or thousands of persons with apparently normal hearing and with no detectable ear disease, preferably young men and women between the ages of 18 and 25, it is possible to find an *average* value for normal hearing. That is to say, we can find the level of sound intensity, at any particular frequency, at which the average person with normal hearing will just barely hear the stimulating tone. But if this level is to be reproduced in all audiometers with reqularity, it is essential for the physicist who designs them and the electronic engineer who makes them to have a fixed and measurable reference level. The physicist measures the intensity of a sound (or more correctly, the *sound pressure*) in terms of newtons per square metre, and the commonly accepted standard reference level for sound pressures is $0.0024 \, \mu N/m^2$. Now, by using this constant reference level, it is possible to fulfil the requirements of any standard—namely, to ensure that tests of the threshold of hearing of a given patient on different audiometers, each complying with this standard, will give substantially the same results under comparable conditions; and that the results obtained will represent a true comparison between the threshold of hearing of the patient and the normal threshold of hearing. The International Standard recommended by the International Standards Organization (ISO) is now in more or less general use, and all audiometers should also be carefully calibrated at regular intervals.

Complex tones – musical sounds, noise and human speech**

It has been said that a pure tone is 'pure' in the sense that it contains only one frequency. But most of the sounds which we normally hear are complex tones—i.e., those which involve simultaneously more than one frequency. And these complex tones derive from musical instruments, from traffic and other noise, and from the organs of human speech.

Musical sounds. The flute and the tuning fork produce almost pure tones. With these and very few other exceptions, nearly all musical instruments produce complex tones, and these can be analysed into their various component pure tones, each with its own frequency and intensity. If the note of middle C is played separately on each of several instruments, the pitch of the note perceived will always be the same – that is to say, it will always be middle C. The pitch will be the same with each instrument because the lowest and the loudest tone in each instance will have the same frequency – 256 Hz. This tone is the *fundamental.*The human ear, however, even without a musical training, can distinguish the tonal qualities of the different instruments; and it is able to do this because each instrument, apart from the fundamental tone which it produces, will also produce a series of *overtones,* most of which are exact and simple multiples of the fundamental – that is, they have frequencies of (for example) two, three and four times that of the basic note. These are harmonic overtones, and it is the presence of these overtones which gives the characteristic tonal quality (or *timbre*) to any particular instrument.

Whatever the instrument, the essential feature common to all *musical* sounds is that their wave-forms all show a regularly repeated pattern (Fig. 3.1, B).

Noise. In contrast to the orderly periodicity of a musical sound, *noise* is distinguished by the random irregularity of its wave-form—that is, by the absence of any repeating pattern. As Professor Dennis Fry has said: 'It is the continuously changing form of the wave motion which causes the hearing mechanism to class the sound as noise'. The extreme example of a continuous noise is one in which high, middle and low frequencies are equally represented and by analogy with the colours of the rainbow, this is known as 'white noise' (Fig. 3.1, C).

A common example of this type of sustained noise is the hissing of escaping steam; but there is another type which consists of a single pulse, such as the sudden back-fire of a motor car.

Human speech. The characteristics of human speech fall somewhere between those of musical sounds and those of noise.

All the vowels and certain consonants (like l, m, and n) have wave-forms like those of musical tones, whilst the consonant sounds of s, f, and sh (like the hissing of steam) are of the nature of sustained noise. P, t and k produce the single-pulse type of noise, whilst many of the voiced consonant sounds (such as b, d, g, z, and v) are mixtures of tone and noise. (D. Fry). The waveform of the simple word TEAS is shown in Fig. 3.1, D (after the late Dr T. S. Littler).

Hearing and speech

We should now be in a position to describe two of the aspects of hearing and speech which are of particular importance to our understanding of the problems of deafness. The first is our ability to hear the many complex sounds of speech; the second, the process by which an infant learns to speck by imitating the speech of those around him. *Hearing for speech.* Voice is produced in the larynx when the air expired by the lungs is forced between the vocal cords under pressure. This causes the cords to vibrate (phonation) as they produce a series of periodic puffs of air, like the lips of a trombone player. This produces the *laryngeal tone,* which is very rich in harmonics and is accompanied by resonances (formants) in the vocal tract above the vocal cords. The fundamental laryngeal tone in men has a frequency of about 125 Hz, in women about 250 Hz; and the sounds used in speech result from modification of these basic laryngeal tones by changes in the shape of throat, mouth and nasal cavities. *Vowels* are continuous sounds, but the *consonants* are produced by putting a sudden check in the course of the expiratory blast of air, by closure of some part or other of the mouth or throat.

Generally speaking, the vowel sounds are lower in frequency than the consonant sounds, and this is shown very well in Fig. 3.4, which I have modified slightly from two excellent graphs prepared and kindly lent to me by my friend and colleague, Dr Mary D. Sheridan.

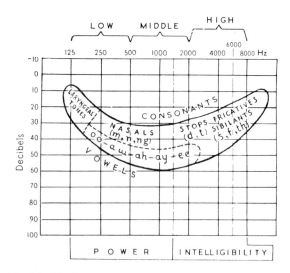

Fig. 3.4   The frequency components of English speech sounds.

In this drawing the sounds used in English speech have been analysed and superimposed on an audiogram. It will be seen that the vowel sound of the lowest frequency is the 'oo' sound (at rather less than 250 Hz); then 'aw' (slightly above 250 Hz); then, in ascending order, 'ah' (about 500 Hz); 'ay' (an octave higher) and 'ee' (at about 2000 Hz). Of the consonant sounds, the nasal sounds (such as m, n, and ng) are the lowest in frequency (about 500 Hz); the fricatives and sibilants (such as s, f and th) the highest (about 6000 Hz). These are produced by the gentle escape of air between the tongue and palate in the first, lower lip and upper teeth in the second, and tongue and upper teeth in the third. Between them lie the stops (such as *d* and *t*), which are produced by a more sudden 'stop' or 'check' to the expiratory air blast between the tongue and the palate.

It must be remembered that (for all voiced sounds) there is, in addition to the components described above, a low-frequency fundamental in the band of frequencies covered by the vibrations of the vocal cords.

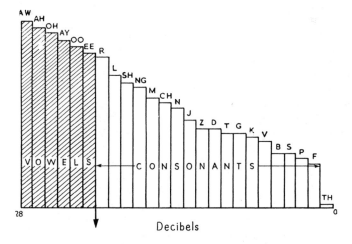

Fig. 3.5   The relative intensities of English speech sounds.

The next drawing (Fig. 3.5) shows that the vowel sounds are not only lower in frequency, but are also higher in intensity, than the consonant sounds. The very faintest sound, for example, is the 'th' sound, which is only just audible at about three feet, and between this and the loudest sound (the vowel sound 'aw') is a difference of nearly 30 dB. Of the vowel sounds, then, it can be said that the sounds 'oo', 'aw' and 'ah' are easy to hear because they are low in pitch and strong in intensity; 'ee', on the other hand, is less easily heard because it is high in pitch and weaker in intensity. And of the consonant sounds, it will be evident that the nasal sounds are relatively easy to hear, whilst the most difficult are the fricative and sibilant sounds.

Why, it may be asked, do we need to know all this? And what is its significance? These questions can best be answered, perhaps, by a simple illustration.

First take a sentence and remove all the consonants. It will look like this:

—e —o— —i- —e —oo— —o— —a— a —o—.

No one can understand it in this form; but it is written and not spoken, and we therefore do not know whether the vowels are long or short. Nevertheless, it helps us very little even if they are given their full value:

ee oh i e uh o ah e ow

It would seem, therefore, that the vowels are relatively unimportant in our comprehension of speech. If this is so, do the consonants alone help us any more? The answer should be apparent as soon as we rewrite the sentence, this time leaving out the vowels:

sh— t–ld h–m th— b–k c–st h–lf – cr–wn

Very soon, if not immediately, its meaning is discernible; and it is no less easy to understand if we use one and the same vowel sound in each and every word:

sher terld herm ther berk cerst herlf er crern.

What does all this amount to? It amounts, quite simply, to this – that, whilst the vowels give power or energy to speech, *intelligibility is provided by the consonants.*

So far we have described only the measurement of hearing for pure tones but it should now be evident that no examination can be regarded as complete until we have some knowledge of hearing for speech. Hearing for the sounds of speech is not, of course, the only factor responsible for understanding. Education and intelligence rank high amongst the others. But it is true, nevertheless, that our ability to hear speech is of the first importance, and it therefore behoves us, in dealing with the deaf patient, to attempt some estimate of his hearing for speech. Live voice tests are used widely with children but they often lack the precision of a standardized test under controlled conditions. In adults and adolescents, however, a more accurate assessment can be made by means of the *speech audiogram.*

Ideally the test should approximate as nearly as possible to hearing for normal conversation; in other words, sentences should be used. But this is so time-consuming that words are more commonly employed. The words should be phonetically balanced—that is to say, they should contain all the phonetic elements (vowels and consonants) of normal speech. The word-list may contain hundreds of words, in phonetically balanced groups of, say, 35 (See Appendix II, p. 225). Each list of 35 words is played from a tape or disc recording at a known intensity, and the person under test listens either through earphones (when each ear can be tested separately) or through a speaker set at a fixed distance from him (free-field speech audiometry). He repeats the words as he hears them, and from his responses a score can be made of the proportion of words (or parts of them) heard correctly. The result is plotted on a graph (Fig. 3.6). This shows the responses that may be expected from a person with normal hearing.

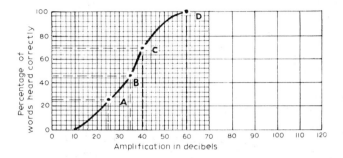

Fig. 3.6   The normal speech audiogram.

The first group of 35 words is played at, say, 25 dB; at this intensity, only one-quarter of the words (25 per cent) are heard correctly (A). Raise the next group of 35 words to an intensity of 35 dB, and he now hears almost one-half of the words (45 per cent) correctly (B). Step up the level of the third group to 40 dB, and the intelligibility score increases rather rapidly to 70 per cent (C). Finally, it will be noted that the person with normal hearing will not hear all the words (100 per cent) correctly until the intensity level reaches a point 60 dB above threshold (D). To express this in a different way. the person with normal hearing should be able to hear everything that is said to him in a normal conversational voice at the usual tete-a-tete distance of about 3 feet.

It should now be evident that two main conditions are necessary for speech to be intelligible; in the first place, the sounds must have an adequate intensity; secondly, an adequate band of frequencies must be present. It has been found experimentally that there is no loss of intelligibility if frequencies below 500 Hz are cut out, and little or nothing is lost by cutting out the frequencies above 4000 Hz. It so happens that this is also the most sensitive range of frequencies for the human ear, and if we can hear these three octaves at an adequate level of intensity, we should be able to hear and understand speech.

Speech through hearing. No child is born with speech. He is born with the instruments of speech—the bellows of the lungs, the wind instrument of the larynx, and the organs of articulation. But the execution of speech is a very complex process—the most highly skilled, in fact, of all forms of motor control. And as a complex series of movements it must be learnt—by a long and arduous process of mimicry—by imitation of the sounds of speech as produced by those around him. And if any of the many complex sounds as speech cannot be heard or otherwise perceived, they cannot and will not be imitated.

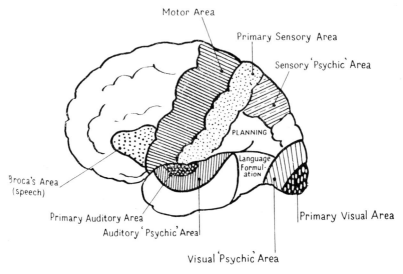

Fig. 3.7   The sensory and motor areas of the brain.

The ear is the normal channel to those areas of the brain which are given over to the development of speech. Sounds have little meaning during the first three months of life and all babies, whether hearing or deaf, vocalize in much the same way in these earliest days. They cry when they are hungry, they gurgle when they are happy and contented. But by the end of the third month the child with normal hearing is beginning to realize that sounds have meaning, and he turns to his mother's voice. From this time onwards, he is seeing and feeling and hearing the people and the objects that surround him, and as these sensations—of sight and feeling and hearing—are reaching the primary centres in the brain, so he is now beginning to associate the sounds emitted by them and the words spoken about them with his own sensations of their appearance and their feel. And little by little, these associations are being stored as memories, in the 'psychic' areas of the brain—those areas which lie in the 'no-man's-land' between the primary areas for sight and touch and hearing (Fig. 3.7). These psychic areas are continually building and storing a mutual understanding of the world about the child, and at the same time he is learning to control the difficult motions of speech.

By the age of 9 months the infant is beginning to sit up and look around him, and by so enlarging his sphere of interest he is becoming, slowly but surely, more and more aware of his surroundings. Throughout the whole of this period between the third and the ninth months of his life, he is learning to distinguish the various sounds about him and to associate them with their source. Not until he has begun to develop this sense of *auditory discrimination* will he make his first attempts at discernible speech, and it is now that he begins to utter his first single syllables. As Dr Sheridan puts it: 'He must listen to the same speech sounds being repeated over and over again before he can store them in his memory, first as phonetic units, then as words with meaning. Only when this process—sensory recognition with intelligent association—is complete can the child repeat the vocal sounds himself with understanding and purpose.' These earliest attempts at definitive speech consist in the first place of vowels only. This is not surprising, of course, for vowel sounds are not only easier to hear, but are also easier to reproduce than the consonants. Nor is it surprising that, at about the time of his first birthday, the first consonants which are added to his ever-growing vocabulary of vowels should be those which are most easily heard and most easily produced—namely, the nasal sounds (such as 'm' and 'n') and the stops (such as 'd' and 't') And so it is that, after a period of almost continuous babbling, with many of the cadences of speech, simple words of two syllables follow and he will now say 'Ma-ma, and 'Da-da'. This first year of life has been described as the *period of readiness for listening* (the late Edith Whetnall).

Those who are closest to him identify themselves with these sounds, and their obvious delight is reflected in the child's re-animated efforts to find new ways of expressing himself. Words begin to take on a new significance and he shows his ability to understand simple commands by responding to them with appropriate actions. Slowly his newly acquired faculty grows, word by word, as he imitates more and more of the sounds that he hears; and he can say about twenty words almost perfectly by the age of 18 months. This first six months of his second year is the natural *period of readiness for speech* (Whetnall). Speech is now well under way: and so it goes on until, by his second birthday, he is putting two or three words together and making short sentences. Thereafter his vocabulary grows with astonishing rapidity, and speech blossoms forth into language.

4. How We Hear – Physiology

Physiology is described as the science of the normal functions and phenomena of living things, and it is the purpose of this chapter to describe the workings of the human ear.

Functionally, the hearing portion of the ear has two parts – a perceiving apparatus which analyses and interprets the sounds which reach it; and a conducting apparatus whose function is simply to carry, or conduct, them to the perceiving apparatus.

The perceiving apparatus consists entirely of neuro-epithelial structures. It begins in the hair-cells of the organ of Corti (the sensory part) and ends in the primary and 'psychic' auditory areas of the brain (the cortical part). Connecting them are the fibres of the auditory nerve (the neural part).

The conducting apparatus consists of the auricle and external auditory canal; the tympanic membrane and the chain of ossicles; the middle ear cleft; and the perilymph and endolymph fluids of the inner ear.

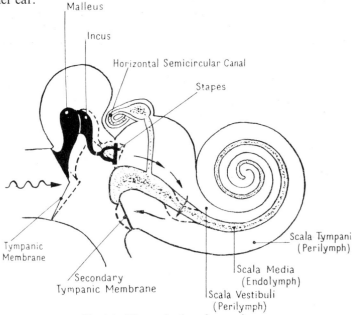

Fig. 4.1   The conduction of a sound wave.

The conduction of sound

Sounds are normally carried to the inner ear by air conduction (AC). They are transmitted across the middle ear cavity, from their source to the oval window, by way of the ossicular chain. This is the most important route, but sound energy may also be taken up and transmitted directly through the bones of the skull, by bone conduction (BC).

The functions of the ossicles (Fig. 4.1) As the alternating compressions and rarefactions of the oncoming sound waves strike the tympanic membrane, it moves in and out. The malleus, attached as it is to the inner surface of the drumhead, moves in and out with it and its movements (together with those of the incus) are transmitted, in turn, to the stapes.

Hence the sound waves collected by the relatively large surface area of the tympanic membrane are carried by the chain of ossicles to the much smaller surface area of the oval window.

The dynamics of the labyrinthine windows

The inward movement of the footplate of the stapes allows the sound waves to travel along the upper gallery of perilymph fluid (scala vestibuli), between the bony and membranous tubes of the cochlea.

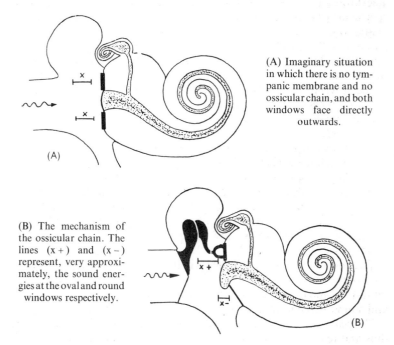

(A) Imaginary situation in which there is no tympanic membrane and no ossicular chain, and both windows face directly outwards.

(B) The mechanism of the ossicular chain. The lines $(x+)$ and $(x-)$ represent, very approximately, the sound energies at the oval and round windows respectively.

Fig. 4.2 The dynamics of the labyrinthine windows.

This fluid movement is transmitted to the endolymph fluid (in the scala media) and so to the lower perilymph gallery (scala tympani).

As the footplate of the stapes moves inwards at the oval window, the secondary tympanic membrane moves outwards at the round window. Were it not for this movement in *opposite phase* of the structures sealing the oval and the round windows, there could be no vibration of the incompressible fluid in the rigid bony labyrinth.

What it is, then, that makes this possible?

By far the most important factor is the preferential distribution of sound energy to the oval window, through the ossicular chain, from the tympanic membrane. If the sound energies at the oval and round windows were equal, no fluid movement would occur in the cochlea (Fig. 4.2, A). But in fact, the greater part of the sound energy applied to the large surface area of the tympanic membrane is transmitted through the ossicular chain to the much smaller surface area of the oval window, and the round window receives only a small fraction of the energy received by the air in the tympanic cavity (Fig. 4.2, B).

The effective areal ratio of the tympanic membrane to the oval window is about 14 to 1; furthermore, the ossicles themselves constitute a lever mechanism, acting through the rotational axis of the malleus and incus, which has a further mechanical advantage of 1.3 to 1. The product of these areal and lever ratios is about 18 to 1, which represents the *transformer ratio* of the whole mechanism. By its mediation, the *amplitude* of vibration at the stapes is reduced as compared with that of the drumhead, whilst the *force* exerted by the stapes upon the labyrinthine fluids is increased in the same proportion. For the maximum transference of acoustic energy from the external air to the labyrinthine fluids, it is essential that the widely differing acoustic impedances (or resistances) of these two media should be 'matched'; and the impedance matching is effected by this *transformer mechanism of the middle ear*.

The transformer system of the ossicular chain results in a 'differential' which works in favour of the oval window.

In addition but to a lesser degree, the differential between the two windows is increased by a difference in elasticity (or texture) of the two windows; by a difference in the angle of incidence of the sound waves upon the closing structures of the windows (see p. 6); and by the sheltering of the round window in its niche by the overhanging promontory.

The effect of the fluid movements in the cochlea is to cause the basilar membrane (together with the organ of Corti mounted upon it) to vibrate up and down, and it is at this point that sound conduction ends and sound perception begins.

Tympanic muscle reflexes. Contraction of the intra-tympanic (stapedius and tensor tympani) muscles increases the stiffness of the middle ear conducting apparatus. They are activated reflexly by sounds of intensities of 90 decibels or above; and by attenuating such loud sounds, especially in the lower frequency range, these reflexes almost certainly protect the inner ear against the effects of excessively loud sounds.

The perception of sound

The cochlea contains the sense-organ of hearing and it is here that sounds are first analysed into their component frequencies, before being passed on to the higher centres in the brain for storage and interpretation.

Stimulation of the organ of Corti. Very slow (sub-sonic) vibrations of the footplate of the stapes will, in theory, produce a flow of peri-lymph up the scala vestibuli, through the helicotrema and down the scala tympani, to the round window membrane, which bulges outwards in opposite phase.

With the rapid vibrations of sound frequencies, however, the acoustic resistance (or impedance) of the inner ear opposes this simple hydraulic effect, and the acoustic energy displaces the organ of Corti and its supporting basilar membrane to and fro between the upper and lower perilymph galleries. It has been shown by von Békésy, a celebrated Nobel laureate, that when the actual vibrations of the basilar membrane are observed, a *travelling wave* (Fig. 4.3) is seen to start from the base of the cochlea and progress towards its apex with increasing amplitude until it reaches an area of maximum displace-

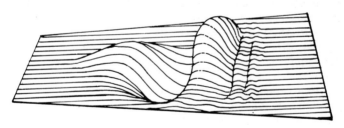

Fig. 4.3 The 'travelling wave' of von Békésy.

ment, the position of which is determined by the frequency of the stimulating tone. Beyond this the wave is rapidly dissipated and disappears. For high frequencies, the maximum displacement of the basilar membrane is confined to the basal turn of the cochlea; low frequencies cause a longer travelling wave, with its maximum ampli-tude near the apex.

Mechanical excitation of the hair-cells. When any particular part of the basilar membrane moves, so does the corresponding unit (or units) of the organ of Corti (which sits upon the membrane) move with it. And as these units move upon the vibrating part of the basilar membrane, there occurs a shearing or sliding movement between the hairs of the hair-cells and the under-surface of the overlying tectorial membrane. This in its turn causes the hairs to be displaced in relation to the bodies of their hair-cells; and it is this motion which produces the so-called 'cochlear microphonic' first described by Wever and Bray and commonly referred to as the Wever-Bray phenomenon. The cochlear microphonics reproduce the frequency and wave-form of the stimulating sound-waves.

Stimulation of the auditory nerve. The exact mechanism by which the fibres of the auditory nerve are stimulated is not known, but it is thought that they may be activated either by the cochlear microphonic, or by the formation or liberation of a chemical substance at the terminations of the nerve fibres in the hair-cells.

Action potential in the auditory nerve. This electrical response represents the sum-total of nervous discharges within the auditory nerve resulting from sound stimulation; and the amplitude of the action potential response gives a fairly good indication of the number of nerve fibres responding to the stimulus.

The subjective attributes of sound

Our subjective sensations of pitch and loudness are dependent, respectively, upon the frequency and intensity of the stimulating tone, and the characteristic timbre (or tone quality) of a complex sound is determined by the frequencies and relative intensities of its component parts; whilst the presence of an ear on each side of the head enables us to localize a sound source.

The analysis of pitch. The two classical theories of pitch analysis are the 'resonance theory' of Helmholtz and the 'telephone theory' of Rutherford.

The 'resonance theory' of Helmholtz

Helmholtz, the great physicist, physician and physiologist, first describe his theory in 1857—in a lecture on the scientific foundations of music.

If the open strings of a piano are exposed to a pure tone of sufficient force, the string whose natural period of vibration (or frequency) corresponds to that of the stimulating tone, will vibrate. It can then be described as a *resonator*.

We have described the basilar membrane as a continuous sheet of tissue supporting a functionally discrete series of some four or five thousand 'units', which together constitute the organ of Corti. Helmholtz conceived of these units as a series of resonators (or 'strings'), each with its own natural period of vibration and each responding only to one tone of one particular frequency. In fact, one could compare them with a series of piano strings. But this idea of a resonating string is too simple for, whereas a piano string vibrates for some time after the driving force has ceased, the ear is 'dead beat' (that is to say, it is critically damped)—or very nearly so. In other words, its movements cease immediately—or within one or two vibrations—after the air has ceased to vibrate.

There is much evidence—anatomical, pathological and experimental —to support Helmholtz's theory.

The frequency of a stretched string is represented by the formula, $F = \frac{1}{2L}\sqrt{\frac{T}{M}}$, where F is the frequency, L is the length, T is the tension, and M is the mass per unit length.

Put in more simple language, the frequency of a stretched string varies directly with its tension and inversely with its length and mass. That is to say, the shorter, lighter and tighter a string is, the higher is the note produced by its vibration.

It has already been said that the four or five thousand 'units' of the organ of Corti can be compared, very broadly, to a series of stretched strings, and it is known that high notes are perceived at the base of the cochlea, low notes at the apex.

In conformity with this, it has been deduced—from the fact that the spiral ligament is more developed at the base than at the apex—that tension is greatest at the base and diminishes towards the apex. Conversely, the length of the basilar membrane is greatest at the apex and least at the base, as also is the mass. These differences in mass are due to 'loading' of the membrane: in the first place, the fluid load of the labyrinthine fluids is greater on the fibres at the apex than at the base, since the columns of fluid are longer; in the second place, fat globules in the cells of Hensen are plentiful at the apex but diminish or disappear towards the base.

Further evidence is provided by the careful study of human pathology and it has been shown, for example, that in cases of high-tone deafness (where the hearing for high tones is grossly affected whilst the hearing for low tones remains good or even normal) atrophic changes have occurred in the organ of Corti and the nerve fibres supplying it at the base of the cochlea.

Finally, electrical potentials generated by low tones are known to arise near the apex of the cochlea, those generated by high tones arising near the base.

According to Helmholtz, therefore, pitch is analysed by the cochlea itself, and the particular nerve fibre which will be stimulated by any particular tone is determined by the particular portion (or 'resonator') of the basilar membrane which is stimulated. Each nerve fibre will carry the impulses to one specific part of the cerebral cortex and, in this way, the basilar membrane is represented in the cortex in a direct point-to-point (or tonotopic) relationship.

The 'telephone theory' of Rutherford

Rutherford was professor of physiology at Edinburgh at the time when he first presented his theory to the public, in a lecture delivered at Birmingham in 1886.

He thought that the basilar membrane vibrated as a whole—like a telephone plate—and he supposed that all the hair-cells throughout the entire organ of Corti would be stimulated by each and every sound, of whatever pitch, and that through those cells the sound-waves were translated into nerve vibrations of corresponding frequency, amplitude and wave-form. Thus, he said, if a pure tone of 440 hertz (Hz) were presented to the ear, the whole basilar membrane would vibrate and electrical charges would travel up the auditory nerve at a rate 440 impulses per second. And if a pure tone of 20 000 Hz were presented to the ear, these impulses would travel up the nerve at the rate of 20 000 per second. According to Rutherford, therefore, pitch was analysed only when these impulses reached the brain.

One of the main difficulties in accepting Rutherford's theory was that he seemed to expect too much of the nerve fibres in the auditory nerve. For although it was known, even in his day, that the human ear could appreciate tones as high as 20 000 Hz, it was known equally well that no nerve fibre (or group of nerve fibres) could conduct electrical impulses at anything like so high a rate. And when in fact, modern physiologists found that the maximum rate of electrical impulses in the auditory nerve was such as to limit the upper frequency of such a system to something less than 1000 Hz, it became evident that Rutherford's theory was not tenable. In fact, neither of the classical theories of pitch perception can fit all the known facts to-day, and just over twenty years ago a third theory—the *volley theory*—was propounded by E. G. Wever.

The 'volley theory' of Wever

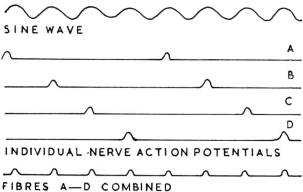

Fig. 4.4   The 'volley theory' of Wever.

In 1949 Wever put forward his volley theory, and it has gained widespread support from its confirmation by subsequent experimental work. He believes that the 'resonance' or 'place' theory of Helmholtz probably accounts for the perception of high frequencies above 5000 Hz, which stimulate the hair-cells only in the basal turn of the cochlea. Furthermore, he believes that the 'telephone' theory of Rutherford probably holds good for the low frequencies, below 400 Hz, which stimulate the whole of the organ of Corti and which are represented in the auditory nerve by action potentials which are directly synchronous with the wave-forms of the applied signals. However, in Wever's opinion, neither of the old theories can account satisfactorily for the perception of tones between 400 Hz and 5000 Hz.

Take a look at Fig. 4.4. The upper tracing represents a sine wave produced by a tone of an intermediate frequency, say 2000 Hz. Now we know that this frequency is far greater than the maximum rate of electrical conductivity in any single nerve fibre. But it will be remembered that the hair-cells connect with the nerve fibres in a complex way, and the middle tracing gives an indication of Wever's idea of what happens when the ear is stimulated by a tone of 2000 Hz. The lines A to D represent four nerve fibres, each of which responds only to every fourth cycle. None of these fibres singly can conduct impulses at the rate of the stimulating tone (shown in the sine wave); but if they are each conducting at different times (that is, asynchronously) in response to the same stimulating tone, the brain will receive, from the combined activity of these four fibres, a synchronous relay of electrical potentials which represent the original frequency of the sine wave. This is shown in the lower tracing. Wever's theory is supported by direct recordings of action potentials in the auditory nerve and in its individual fibres.

The recognition of several pitches

So far we have discussed only the mechanism whereby the cochlea is able to analyse single pure tones. But, as John Mills reminds us in his book *A Fugue in Cycles and Bels,* if the ear were not able to respond to more than one sound wave at a time, 'There would be neither music nor speech as we now know them'.

What happens, then, when we listen to tones of many different pitches, as in orchestral music or speech? 'So far as can be judged by experiment,' says Professor Hartridge, 'the ear has the ability of enabling a listener to recognize the presence of every one of these tones independently of the rest. ... Thus each tone is recognized as if it alone were present. Presumably this means that each tone sets into vibration its own particular part of the basilar membrane. This is followed by the stimulation of a particular part of the brain, and the interpretation of the sounds as a whole automatically follows.'

The recognition of tonal quality (timbre)

It is the ability on the part of the ear to recognize several pitches at one and the same time that allows us to distinguish one musical instrument (or one voice) from another (see page 19). If, for example, a pianist plays the note of A (440 Hz), we can hear not only the fundamental (with a frequency of 440 Hz) but also several overtones (with frequencies which are simple multiples of the fundamental). If a violinist now plays the same note we can also recognize the fundamental tone and several overtones. In both cases the note will sound to us like the note of A (440Hz) because the fundamental in each instance will be the same, and this fundamental is the loudest tone in any complex mixture of tones. But we have no difficulty in saying that the first note A has been played on a piano, the second note A on a violin; and these differences in the quality or timbre of different musical instruments are due to the simultaneous recognition by the listener of the different overtones which accompanied the fundamental tone, and by the assessment of the relative intensities of the overtones in comparison with the fundamental and with one another.

The appreciation of loudness. The sensation of loudness is determined partly by the number of auditory nerve fibres which are activated by the stimulating sound, and partly by the number of impulses carried by each fibre.

The localization of sound. It is usually a fairly simple matter to localize the source of a sound if it comes directly from one or other side of the listener, and its direction is determined partly by the difference in loudness perceived by the two ears, and partly by the difference in the time of reception by the two ears. To a lesser extent it is also possible to say whether a sound comes from directly behind or directly in front. In such an event the sound will, of course, arrive simultaneously at each ear and the sensation of loudness will be the same in both. But the presence of the auricles will screen some of the higher tones from those sounds which come from behind, and it is the difference in the resultant quality of the sound which enables us to say whether it comes from behind or in front.

5. Conductive and Sensori-neural (Perceptive) Deafness

Just as the physiologist describes the ear as consisting functionally of two parts—a conducting apparatus and a perceiving apparatus—so the otologist describes two main types of deafness—conductive and perceptive (sensorineural).

Conductive deafness is caused by any affection of the conducting apparatus—the external auditory canal, the middle ear cleft, or the labyrinthine windows.

Sensori-neural deafness is caused by any affection of the perceiving apparatus—the cochlea (sensory) or the auditory nerve (neural).

To these we can add a third type—*Mixed deafness.* This term is usually applied to a mixture of conductive and perceptive deafness occurring in one and the same ear.

The subjective clinical characteristics of conductive and sensori-neural deafness

The first step in the diagnosis of deafness is to find out whether it is conductive or sensori-neural in type, and a careful history will often take us some way towards this goal.

Perhaps the most characteristic feature of conductive deafness is the *paracusis* of Willis, which occurs particularly in otosclerosis (see page 97).

Thomas Willis lived in the seventeenth century and he carried on a large medical practice in London. Among his several contributions to the scientific literature of his day was a book called *De Anima Brutorum,* published in 1672, and it was in this work that he first described his 'paracusis'—the ability to hear better in noisy surroundings than in quiet surroundings. 'I heard from a credible person,' he writes, 'that he once knew a woman, though she were deaf, yet so long as a drum was beaten within her chamber, she heard every word perfectly: wherefore her husband kept a drummer on purpose for his servant, that by that means he might have some converse with his wife!'

The exact mechanism of paracusis is not known with certainty, but the simplest explanation may account for it in part. The patient with conductive deafness will nearly always hear and understand speech provided that we make it loud enough. In a quiet room, those of us who have normal hearing speak softly and the patient has difficulty in hearing what we say. In a noisy atmosphere, we raise our voices unconsciously and it is partly because our speech is louder that the patient with conductive deafness, untroubled by the background noise, hears it better. However, this alone cannot account for the phenomenon of paracusis; for if this were so, every patient with a conductive deafness should hear better in noisy than in quiet surroundings. Yet it is known that it occurs much more commonly in otosclerosis than in other affections of the conducting apparatus; and it has been suggested that the continuous presence of noise in the background, as in a moving vehicle or a factory or a noisy restaurant, 'sensitizes' the conducting mechanism in such a way that it becomes more receptive to the sounds of speech within that environment.

But the patient with sensori-neural deafness reacts quite differently. He is deafened, not helped, by noise. To him, a sound of low intensity may be barely audible, but a relatively slight increase in the *intensity* of the sound is accompanied by an enormously increased sensation of *loudness*. A point may be reached, indeed, when the subjective sensation of loudness experienced by the patient equals or exceeds that experienced by the person with normal hearing.

This is the *loudness recruitment phenomenon*, described by the late E.P. Fowler in 1936.

As the sensation of loudness increases with abnormal rapidity, the recruiting patient can tolerate only a slight increase in the intensity. of speech. But a sudden and rapid increase does, in fact, occur very often in normal speech, and the difference between the faintest and the loudest speech sounds within a single short sentence may be as great as 30 decibels (see page 21). This causes distortion and discomfort. The patient asks us not to shout.

Furthermore, in cases of sensori-neural deafness, the hearing loss for high tones is characteristically greater than for low tones and, if we speak too rapidly, the soft high-pitched consonant sounds of speech are swamped by the waves of loud low-pitched vowels. Intelligibility suffers and we are asked to speak slowly.

Paracusis occurs only in a limited proportion of cases of conductive deafness, recruitment only in certain types of sensori-neural deafness. Their absence, therefore, does not exclude that particular type of deafness with which each is commonly associated. But the presence of either of these features is so highly characteristic as to be almost diagnostic.

The patient's voice may give us a further hint as to the nature of his deafness. Normally we regulate the loudness of our voices by the way in which we ourselves hear them. And we hear our own voices partly by bone conduction, partly by air conduction. The patient with a conductive deafness will hear his own voice less well by air conduction, but relatively better by bone conduction; and he may feel that he is shouting when, in fact, he is talking normally. He therefore tends to lower his voice. This applies particularly to the otosclerotic, whose faint speech may be almost inaudible, especially in noisy surroundings.

In contrast with this, the patient with a sensori-neural deafness hears his own voice (as everything else) less well by bone conduction, and for this reason he will commonly feel that he is not talking loudly enough. Everyone must be familiar with the harsh, loud raucous voice of the old man whose cochlea is wearing out.

6. The Functional Examination of Hearing

The final distinction between conductive and sensori-neural deafness depends upon the functional examination of the patient's hearing. Many methods are available.

Voice and whisper tests

Applied as single words or short sentences, live voice and whisper tests are of very limited value as standardization is impossible and, even with the same examiner, the intensity of spoken or whispered sounds varies from day to day—even from hour to hour—and under different acoustic conditions. At best, therefore, these tests can provide only a rough idea of the patient's hearing, and they add little information to that already gained by the taking of a history.

Turning fork tests

It is nearly always possible, in adults, to distinguish a pure conductive deafness from a pure sensori-neural deafness by the careful performance of two or three simple tuning fork tests.

The fork most commonly used for standard testing has a frequency of either 256 Hz (Fig. 6.1) or 512 Hz. If a fork of too low a frequency is used, it becomes difficult to distinguish hearing from vibration; and if one of too high a frequency is used, it fades too quickly.

It must be possible to hold the tuning fork firmly by its stem without interfering with its vibrations, and its base must be flat, and broad enough to be applied to the mastoid process. If the fork is struck too forcibly, overtones may become prominent and the test invalidated thereby.

Hearing by bone conduction can be regarded as a rough clinical measure of perceptive function and, provided that this is normal, hearing by air conduction will give us a rough guide to the integrity—or otherwise—of the conducting mechanism.

Weber's test. E. H. Weber of Leipzig first described his test, as it is known and practised today, in 1834. It was the first of the standard tuning fork tests still in current use.

The fork is struck lightly and its base is placed anywhere in the midline of the skull—usually and preferably on the forehead.

Weber's test is used mainly in cases of unilateral deafness, and the patient is asked to say in which ear he hears the fork.

Hearing by bone conduction is reduced in disorders of the perceiving mechanism and the fork is therefore heard less well in the affected ear than in the normal ear in cases of unilateral sensori-neural deafness. The Weber response is then said to be referred to the normal ear.

On the other hand, hearing by bone conduction remains normal in disorders of the conducting mechanism, whilst hearing by air conduction is reduced. And it is this reduced hearing by air conduction which causes the fork to be heard better in the affected ear than in the normal ear in cases of unilateral conductive deafness. The explanation is as follows: under normal conditions of clinical testing, there is a considerable level of background noise; this ambient noise (as it is called) reaches the ears by air conduction, and it *masks* the sound of the tuning fork as heard by bone conduction; in the normal ear, hearing by air conduction is normal and the masking effect of ambient noise is therefore maximal; in the affected ear hearing by air conduction is reduced and the masking effect of the ambient noise is therefore less. Consequently, the normal ear will cease to hear the fork some time before its last vibrations have died away. But the affected ear will hear it longer—and louder. Hence the Weber response is referred to the the affected ear.

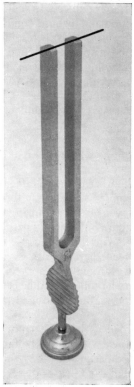

Fig. 6.1 Tuning fork (256 Hz). (*Down Bros. and Mayer and Phelps.*) The 'acoustic axis' is indicated by the black line.

Rinne's test. Adolf Rinne of Göttingen described in 1855 the test which bears his name. Each ear is tested separately.

The tuning fork is struck lightly and its base is held on the mastoid process of the ear under test. After one or two seconds, it is transferred to the opening of the external auditory canal, with its acoustic axis (Fig. 6.1) in line with the axis of the canal. The fork is held alternately on the mastoid process and at the ear, until it is no longer heard by one or the other.

In the normal subject the fork is heard about twice as long by air conduction as by bone conduction, and this normal relationship (AC > BC) is described as a positive Rinne response.

In cases of sensori-neural deafness, the hearing of bone conduction is reduced. So also is the hearing by air conduction, but to a lesser extent. The normal relationship (AC > BC) is therefore retained and the Rinne test is still positive.

In cases of conductive deafness, the hearing by bone conduction remains normal, whilst hearing by air conduction is reduced. In slighter degrees of deafness, the hearing by air conduction and by bone conduction may be equal (AC = BC), and the Rinne response is then said to be *neutral*. But a point is soon reached where the hearing by air conduction is reduced below the hearing by bone conduction, and this reversal in the normal relationship (AC < BC, or more commonly BC > AC) is known as a *negative* Rinne response.

The *false negative Rinne response* is found in cases of severe unilateral sensorineural deafness.

Suppose, for example, that a patient has a total unilateral sensorineural deafness in his right ear. Strike a tuning fork and hold it at the opening of the right (deaf) external auditory canal. If it is struck lightly—as it should be—it will not be heard, either in the right ear or in the left (normal) ear, because the attenuation (or reduction in force) of air-conducted sound between the two ears is very great (about 55 dB).

But if the fork is now transferred to the right (deaf) mastoid process it will almost certainly be heard in the left (normal) ear, because the attentuation of bone-conducted sound between the two ears is very small (only about 5–10 dB). This patient, however, may not appreciate that he is hearing the fork in his normal ear and he will say that he hears the fork when it is applied to his mastoid process, but not outside the ear, on the affected side.

Such a result should, of course, be recorded as BC only—not as BC > AC—and the false negative Rinne response will usually be fairly obvious to anyone who is familiar with it, especially as the Weber response will usually be referred to the normal ear in cases of severe unilateral sensori-neural deafness. But it can be very easily overlooked if the examiner is not aware of its existence and I have seen several cases in which failure to recognize the false negative response led to an erroneous diagnosis of conductive deafness—including one case of auditory nerve tumour in which a fatal outcome might have been avoided if the true nature of the deafness had been recognized early enough.

Masking. The final distinction between a false negative and a true negative Rinne response is made by *'masking'* the normal ear with a Bárány noise box while the test is repeated in the deaf ear. The Bárány box (Fig. 6.2) has a simple clockwork mechanism which produces 'white noise' (see page 19). Held close to the normal ear, it prevents that ear from hearing the sounds of the tuning fork when the fork is applied to the mastoid process on the affected side.

The absolute bone conduction test. The ABC test is a test of perceptive function in which the patient's hearing by bone conduction is compared

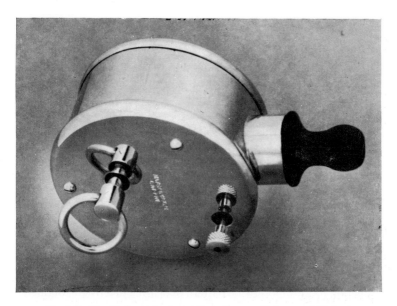

Fig. 6.2   The Bárány noise box. (*Down Bros. and Mayer and Phelps.*)

with the examiner's

The masking effects of ambient noise have been described in the account of Weber's test, and it is the exclusion of hearing by air conduction which makes this test of bone conduction *absolute*. This is achieved, for clinical purposes, by occluding the external auditory canal of the ear under test with the examiner's finger. The patient's hearing by bone conduction is first determined by placing the base of the tuning fork on his mastoid process. Next, the examiner, occluding his own canal in the same way, transfers the fork to his own mastoid process and compares his own ability to hear it with the patient's. If the examiner can still hear the fork after the patient has ceased to hear it, then the patient's absolute bone conduction is said to be reduced. And a reduction in the patient's ABC will usually indicate a sensorineural deafness.

The results of the standard tuning fork tests can best be summarized in tabular form.

	Weber's Test	Rinne's Test	ABC Test
Conductive Deafness	BC referred to deaf ear	Negative (BC > AC)	ABC normal
Sensori-neural Deafness	BC referred to normal ear	Positive (AC > BC) (False negative (BC only, in severe unilateral sensori-neural deafness)	ABC reduced

Despite the great technical advances of the last half-century, these simple tuning-fork tests still hold an important place in the qualitative assessment of deafness in adults.

Other tuning-fork tests may be used in the detection of non-organic hearing loss, and these are described in Chapter 19.

Pure tone audiometry

The principles and technique of pure tone audiometry have been described briefly in Chapter 3 (page 16), and it remains here only to discuss the characteristic audiometric features of conductive and sensori-neural deafness.

Conductive deafness. There is usually a greater loss of hearing by air conduction for low tones than for high tones in the slighter degrees of conductive deafness (Fig. 6.3, A). The curve tends to flatten as the deafness progress (Fig. 6.3, B), but in advanced cases in which sensori-neural deafness may tend to supervene, the loss may be greater for high tones (Fig. 6.3, C).

In cases of conductive deafness, the pattern of hearing loss by bone conduction follows closely the pattern of hearing loss by air conduction but, whatever the extent of the loss, the hearing by bone conduction remains better than the hearing by air conduction (negative Rinne response).

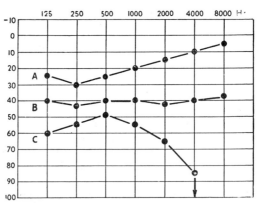

Fig. 6.3   Pure tone audiograms in typical cases of
conductive deafness (air conduction only).
A, Slight.   B, Moderate.   C, Severe.

Sensori-neural deafness. One of the characteristic features of sensori-neural deafness is that the air-conducted hearing for high tones tends to be affected earlier than the hearing for low tones (Fig. 6.4, A). (One notable exception to this 'rule' is to be found in early cases of Menière's disease). This tendency may be maintained at any stage of perceptive deafness (Fig. 6.4, C), but the audiogram may flatten as it advances

(Fig. 6.4, B).

Bone conduction measurements are open to many objections in pure tone audiometry, and it may not be possible to demonstrate the positive Rinne response (AC > BC) on the audiogram. But the shape of the bone conduction audiogram will usually follow that of the air conduction curve and the amount of loss by bone conduction in cases of sensori-neural deafness will always be below that of the normal threshold response, because hearing by bone conduction gives a measure of perceptive function.

Severe unilateral sensori-neural deafness

The false negative Rinne response has been described on page 40, and further difficulty may arise in cases of severe unilateral sensori-neural deafness when pure tone audiometry is used.

Suppose again that we are examining a patient who has a total deafness in his right ear, with normal hearing in the left. Theoretically, we should expect to obtain a normal audiogram in the left ear, with no response in the right. In fact, however, a *'shadow curve'* is produced on the affected side, parallel to the normal audiogram but at a level of about 55 dB below it (Fig. 6.5, A and B).

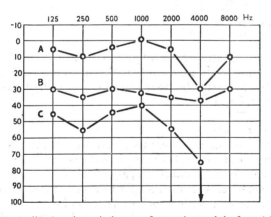

Fig. 6.4 Pure tone audiograms in typical cases of sensori-neural deafness (air conduction only).   A, Slight. B, Moderate. C, Severe.

Masking in pure tone audiometry

As already explained, the attenuation of air-conducted sound between the two ears is in the region of 55 dB, and it is for this reason that a pure tone applied to the totally deafened (right) ear will be heard at this intensity. But it is, of course, being heard in the normal (left) ear, although this may not be recognized by the patient. In any case in which the difference in hearing loss between the two ears is 55 dB or greater, the test must therefore be repeated by masking the better ear with 'white noise' (see page 40) while the testing tone is re-applied to the worse ear. Such a masking noise can be produced by the audiometer and its intensity should be about 45 dB below that of the test tone. The effect of such masking is to increase the threshold intensity level in the worse ear (Fig. 6.5, C).

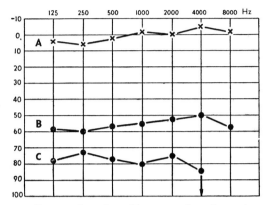

Fig.6.5   Pure tone audiogram of a patient with severe unilateral sensori-neural deafness (air conduction only).
A, Left ear—normal hearing.
B, Right ear—unmasked—'shadow curve'.
C, Right ear—left ear 'masked'.

(Because the attenuation of bone-conducted sound is very small —only about 5 or 10 dB—masking (by air conduction) should *always* be used when hearing by bone conduction is being measured by pure tone audiometry.)

Recruitment of loudness

The phenomenon of loudness recruitment was first recorded in certain cases of unilateral perceptive deafness and its subjective clinical features have been described on page 36.

For several years it was thought to occur in every case of sensori-neural deafness, but the work of Dix, Hallpike, and Hood in this country cast considerable early doubts on the veracity of this opinion and it is now generally believed that it is present only in cases of sensory deafness due to affections of the organ of Corti (end-organ deafness). It is absent or incomplete in neural deafness due to affections of the nerve, and it never occurs in conductive deafness.

Several methods now exist for the detection of loudness recruitment.

(i) *Alternate binaural loudness balance.* The test originally described by Fowler was applied to cases of unilateral deafness and is known as the alternate binaural loudness balance test—'binaural' because a comparison is made between the deaf ear and the normal ear; 'alternate' because the testing tone is presented alternately to each ear; and 'loudness balance test' because the subject under test is asked to balance the sensation of loudness experienced in the two ears.

A single pure tone, commonly of 1000 Hz, is used and it is now customary to deliver this tone to each ear separately, either through two separate audiometers or through a single audiometer with two independent oscillators. The result is plotted on a graph (Fig. 6.6).

The curve A represents the result that is to be expected in a person with normal hearing. If the hearing is normal in both ears, the threshold should be 0 dB in each (A.1). Now present the same tone (of 1000 Hz) to the right ear at an intensity of 20 dB above this threshold and ask the subject to note the degree of loudness which he experiences. Then present the tone to the left ear at the same intensity and the sensation of loudness will be the same. Hence an equal sensation of *loudness* will be experienced in the two ears when the *intensity* of the stimulating tone is equal (20 dB). This gives the point A.2. By repeating the mea-

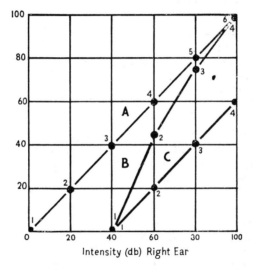

Fig. 6.6   Binaural loudness balance test. *(E. P. Fowler)*. A, Normal response.   B, Recruiting deafness.   C, Non-recruiting deafness.

surements in steps of 20 dB (at 40, 60, 80 and 100 dB) one finds that a constant relationship between intensity and loudness is maintained (A. 3, 4, 5, and 6). The resultant graph is a straight line at 45 degrees.

The curve B represents the result that is obtained in the patient with a 'recruiting' deafness. His pure tone audiogram shows a hearing loss of 40 dB in the right ear. Since the pure tone audiogram gives us a threshold measurement and since the hearing in the left ear is normal, the sensation of loudness experienced by the right (deaf) ear at an intensity of 40 dB is the same as that experienced by the left (normal) ear at 0 dB (B. 1). Increase the intensity of the stimulating tone in the the right ear to 60 dB and ask the patient to balance the sensation of loudness with that in his left ear. This occurs when the intensity of the stimulating tone in the normal ear reaches, say, 45 dB (B. 2). Further points are plotted at intensities (for the deaf ear) of 80 dB and 100 dB and above this level if necessary—and the effect of balancing the sensation of loudness experienced at these levels will be seen at B.3 and B.4. It will be evident that the *difference* in intensity between the stimulating tones at the deaf and the normal ear diminishes as the actual intensity at the deaf ear increases. The gap has narrowed, the curve for the deaf ear has approached and met that of the normal ear, and loudness has 'recruited'. This is the sort of result that is to be expected in the patient with a unilateral deafness of the sensory (or end-organ) type.

The curve C shows the loudness balance graph of patient with a unilateral conductive deafness. As in the former example, his right ear shows a loss of 40 dB on the pure tone audiogram and this threshold response is balanced by an intensity of 0 dB in the left ear (C.1). The same tone is now presented to the deaf ear at intensities of 60, 80, and 100 dB, and the sensation of loudness in his deaf ear is balanced by an equal sensation of loudness in the normal ear at intensities of 20, 40, and 60 dB (C.2, 3 and 4). The *difference* in intensity between the stimulating tones at the deaf ear and the normal ear remains constant—it is always 40 dB. The 'curve' is therefore a straight line parallel to the normal curve A and there is no recruitment of loudness.

Hence it may be possible to distinguish a conductive from a sensorineural deafness by the alternate binaural loudness balance test, but its application is limited by the fact that its use is confined to cases of unilateral deafness, or to cases in which there is a difference of at least 30 dB between the ears.

(ii) *Difference limen for intensity (Békésy)*. Because of the limitations of Fowler's test, many attempts have been made to devise one which can be applied equally well to cases of unilateral and of bilateral deafness. Most of them depend upon measurements of the *minimum perceptible difference* (MPD) of loudness—that is to say, we must determine what changes in the *intensity* of various stimulating tones will be required to effect a change in the *sensation of loudness* which is only just detectable by the listener. In terms of audiometry this minimum perceptible difference is known as the *Difference Limen for intensity* (DL).

Many DL tests have come and gone and none can claim to be wholly reliable, but the one described by Békésy is perhaps the most firmly established.

Békésy audiometry

In discussing the loudness recruitment phenomenon in the previous chapter it has been said that a relatively slight increase in the intensity of a stimulating sound is accompanied by a *relatively* great increase in the subjective sensation of loudness. It follows from this that the amount of increase in intensity that will be required to produce a difference in the sensation of loudness will be less in the recruiting patient than in the normal subject. This is the basis of Békésy's test.

The Békésy audiometer produces, in its simplest original form, a continuous auditory stimulus whose frequency is automatically raised from bottom to top of the testing range, at a very slow rate. As the patient listens to the changing tones he himself controls their intensity with a press button, and his adjustments are recorded by a small pen on an audiograph which moves round with the changing frequencies. He is asked to press the button as soon as he hears a tone. This automatically engages a motor-driven attenuator which reduces the intensity of the tone until it disappears below the patient's threshold. At this point he releases the button and the intensity of the tone is automatically raised again. In this way the patient traces his own audiogram which tells us when he just hears a sound and when he just ceases to hear it. Two results are shown in Fig. 6.7. The variability in the threshold of hearing is shown by the length of the excursions above and below the average threshold and this variability gives us a measure of the difference limen.

The graph A shows the Békésy audiogram of a patient who does not recruit. The variations around the average threshold are about 10–15 dB from peak to trough and are of roughly the same order as occur in the normal listener. The graph B, on the other hand, shows the audiogram of a recruiting patient. Here it will be noted that variations (of DL) around the average threshold diminish as the hearing loss gradually increases above a frequency of between 500 and 1000 Hz.

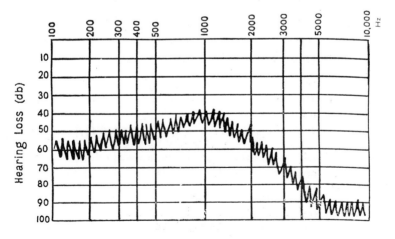

(A)   Non-recruiting deafness.

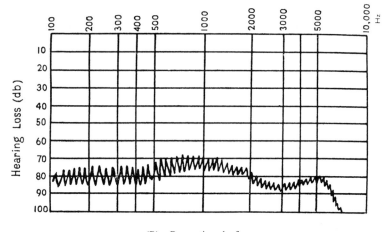

(B)   Recruiting deafness.

Fig. 6.7   Békésy audiogram.

J. Jerger has shown that it is possible to obtain further information about the site of a lesion if the patient is presented not only with a continuous sound, but also with an interrupted sound which is pulsed rapidly on and off. The relationship between the two tracings allows us to classify Békésy audiographs into five types (Fig. 6.8), whereby it may be possible to distinguish a sensory from a neural deafness.

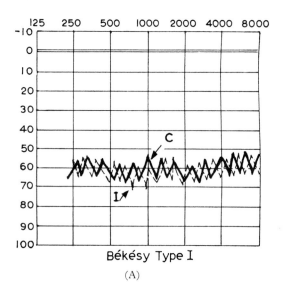

Békésy Type I

(A)

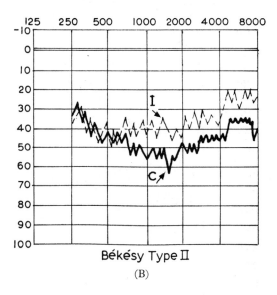

Békésy Type II

(B)

Fig. 6.8 Jerger's types of Békésy audiographs.

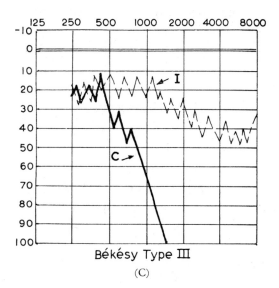

Békésy Type III

(C)

In type I, the continuous ('C') tracing overlaps the interrupted ('I') tracing (Fig. 6.8, A). Both are about 10 dB wide. It occurs in normal ears or in conductive hearing losses.

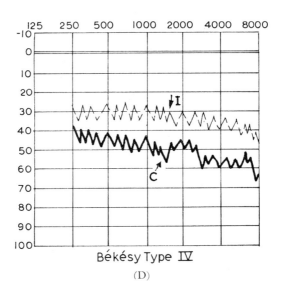

Békésy Type IV

(D)

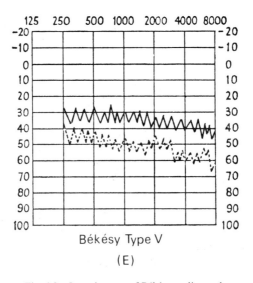

Békésy Type V

(E)

Fig. 6.8   Jerger's types of Békésy audiographs.

In type II, the 'C' tracing overlaps the 'I' tracing (Fig. 6.8, B) in the low frequencies, but at some point between 500 and 1000 Hz, it drops 10–15 dB below the 'I' tracing and retains that position up to the highest frequencies. It occurs only when the disorder is in the cochlea, but not in every cochlear lesion.

In type III, the 'C' tracing drops dramatically below the 'I' tracing (Fig. 6.8, C), sometimes as much as 40–50 dB. The break may occur at any point in the frequency range, and once the 'C' tracing begins to drop, it usually continues downwards. This type of graph is typical of neural deafness and indicates severe *tone decay*, a phenomenon in which there is a progressive elevation of the auditory threshold for a continuous pure tone.

In type IV, the 'C' tracing runs well below the 'I' tracing at *all* frequencies (Fig. 6.8, D). This is more common in neural than in sensory deafness.

In type V, the 'C' tone is heard better than the pulsed 'I' tone. It is always suggestive of a non-organic hearing loss.

Carhart's test

This is another test of *tone decay* (see reference to Type III Jerger tracing, above). A tone is presented continuously at 5 dB above the subjective threshold, for 60 seconds. If the subject ceases to hear this tone, the intensity is increased without break by another 5 dB. The test is continued until the subject is able to hear the tone for 30 seconds, or until a maximum of 3 minutes has elapsed from the start of the test.

In normal subjects and those with conductive hearing losses, there is a decay of 0–15 dB; in sensory deafness, the decay is of the order of 0–20 dB; and in neural deafness it exceeds 20 dB.

Short increment sensitivity index (SISI) test

Many patients with disorders of the cochlea are able to detect smaller changes in sound intensity than those with normal hearing or those with affections of the VIIIth nerve or middle ear. This forms the basis of the SISI test, and it is really a simplification of the original Békésy test.

The ear under test is presented with a continuous pure tone, usually beginning at 1000 Hz, always at 20 dB above threshold. Every five seconds, the intensity jumps by an extra 1 dB for a period of three-tenths of a second. Some of these increments are heard, some are not; but the patient is asked to press a button each time he experiences an increase in loudness. This is repeated for 20 jumps, and the patient's score is the percentage of increments heard correctly. The test may be given at any frequency, but it is usually confined to those between 250 Hz and 4000 Hz.

Persons with normal hearing, or those with affections of the middle

ear or VIIIth nerve, usually score between 0 and 20 per cent at all frequencies. Positive scores (60–100 per cent) occur only in patients with
cochlear disorders, such as Menière's disease or acoustic trauma.
Even in these cases, however, high SISI scores tend to occur only at
frequencies above 1000 Hz.

Loudness discomfort level
   The level of sound which causes discomfort to the patient is measured.
This loudness discomfort level (LDL) is normally reached in subjects
with normal hearing at a level of 90–105 dB, and in patients with
conductive or neural deafness, the maximum output of the audiometer
(up to 120 dB) is usually well tolerated; in recruiting deafness, intensities of less than 80 dB above the patient's threshold may cause considerable discomfort.

The site of the lesion
   The intelligent application of these tests of loudness recruitment
enables the otologist, in many instances, to locate the site of a lesion
producing a sensorineural deafness. When the deafness affects one
ear only, the alternate binaural loudness balance test of Fowler is by
far the most accurate. It will show evidence of partial or complete
recruitment in affections of the cochlear end-organ, such as Menière's
disease or acoustic trauma; but no recruitment occurs in affections of
the auditory (VIIIth) nerve, such as a tumour.
   Békésy audiometry, Carhart's test and measurement of the loudness
discomfort level are of particular value in cases of bilateral perceptive
deafness. In lesions of the end-organ, there is a Type II tracing in the
Békésy audiogram and tone decay is minimal; in lesions of the auditory
nerve, the Békésy audiogram shows a Type III or Type IV tracing and
tone decay is marked.
   Many other tests are under trial, and new ones are being constantly
developed; but they are all extremely time-consuming, and these
three are now so well established as to give invaluable information in
many obscure cases of nerve deafness.

The physiology of loudness recruitment
   Three main theories have been advanced to explain the phenomenon
of loudness recruitment.
   In the first of these, recruitment is assumed to depend upon the fact
that each fibre of the cochlear nerve makes contact not only with one
hair-cell but with several, and that each hair-cell makes contact not
only with one nerve fibre, but with several; and the inner hair-cells
receive many times more fibres than the outer hair-cells. Hence, it is
argued, if a sound of weak intensity is applied to a deafened ear in
which the hair-cells are damaged, the stimulation of outer hair-cells
will be sufficient to activate only a *few* of the nerve fibres which innervate

them. The sensation of loudness experienced by the deafened ear will therefore be less than in the normal ear. However, if the sound is of very strong intensity, the stimulation of the inner hair-cells will be able to 'saturate' *all* of the nerve fibres which innervate them. Hence the sensation of loudness experienced by the deafened ear will be the same as that in the normal ear.

In the second theory, it is suggested that recruitment may be accounted for by a difference in sensitivity of the outer and inner hair-cells, the outer hair-cells responding to both loud and faint sounds, the inner hair-cells being stimulated only by loud sounds. When the more vulnerable *outer* hair-cells are damaged, the cochlea will not respond at threshold intensities, but the *inner* hair-cells, which retain their normal sensitivity, will be stimulated by louder sounds.

At very high intensities, the deafened ear may hear the sound louder than the normal ear (over-recruitment). A neural 'feedback' circuit may exist whereby the output of the outer hair-cells inhibits the output of the inner hair-cells; and loss of the outer hair-cells may damage this mechanism, with the result that the output of the inner hair-cells is unchecked.

Speech audiometry

The main objection to pure tone audiometry is that it may give us little or no idea of the patient's ability to hear and *understand* speech, and no test of hearing can be said to be complete until we have made some attempt to assess this particular faculty.

A crude quantitative assessment of speech intelligibility can be made by measuring the distance at which set words or sentences can be repeated. But the examiner's voice will tend to vary from day to day and it is therefore difficult to compare the results of such 'free-field' testing on two or more separate occasions. This can be obviated to some extent by 'monitoring' the speech with a sound level meter which measures the intensity of the speech sounds at the level of the ear being tested. For more accurate measurements, however, the patient's ability to hear and understand speech is best determined by speech audiometry.

The principles of speech audiometry have been described in the chapter on acoustics, but apart from giving us a quantitative measure of speech intelligibility, the speech audiogram will also disclose certain qualitative differences which allow us to distinguish a conductive from a sensorineural deafness (Fig. 6.9).

Imagine that we have two patients, X and Y, each with a hearing loss by air-conduction of 60 dB, as measured on the pure tone audiometer.

The patient X has a severe conductive deafness. His curve is parallel to that of the normal hearing person (N) but is shifted to the right; that is to say, words must be spoken much more loudly to make him hear them as well as the person with normal hearing. He will be able to hear 50 per cent of the words correctly, for example, only at an intensity of about 95 dB; and he will not hear all the words correctly until the intensity is raised to about 120 dB. But the important point is this: that if sounds can be made loud enough, the patient with a pure conductive deafness can usually be made to hear speech normally or almost normally.

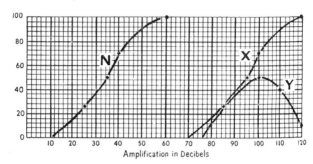

Fig. 6.9 The speech audiograms of conductive and sensori-neural deafness. N, Normal response. X, Conductive deafness. Y, Sensori-neural deafness.

The patient Y has a severe sensori-neural deafness. Even at an intensity of 100 dB, he is able to hear only 50 per cent of words correctly. But worse still, if the intensity is now raised to 110 dB, he will understand even less—only 40 per cent—and he will, in fact, never be able to understand everything that is said to him through hearing alone. Amplification will improve his speech intelligibility up to a certain point, but beyond that point intelligibility decreases as amplification increases. This type of curve (the parabola) is never found in pure conductive deafness, and it has been said that this sort of response is characteristic of the recruiting patient and is therefore found in patients with sensory deafness. Characteristically, very poor scores are achieved in cases of neural deafness.

Be that as it may, the speech audiogram gives us an invaluable overall picture and is, at one and the same time, a reliable qualitative and quantitative test of hearing.

Objective audiometry

It will be evident that all the forms of audiometry so far described must depend, for accurate results, upon the willing co-operation of the person under test to make known his own subjective reactions to a variety of testing sounds. Unfortunately, such co-operation is not always forthcoming, especially in very young or disturbed children, in malingerers, or in adult sufferers from deafness of emotional origin; and it is for just such cases that many attempts have been made to develop some form of truly objective audiometry which will overcome these difficulties.

Impedance measurements

A low-frequency signal or probe tone (for example, 220 Hz) is introduced into the sealed external auditory canal. If the tympanic membrane is immobile (as in fixation of the stapes due to otosclerosis), more of the sound is impeded than when the tympanic membrane is mobile, i.e. compliant (as in disconnexion of the ossicular chain due, for example, to head injury).

The amount of sound reflected is monitored by a sound pressure level meter.

Tympanometry. This was first described by Terkildsen and Thomsen in 1959. The drumhead may be made stiffer, artificially, by changing the air pressure in the external auditory canal, from − 400 mm water pressure to + 200 mm water pressure, by using a small air-pump attached to a manometer. Changes in acoustic impedance are shown by the meter needle, or plotted automatically against the pressure changes on a graph.

The compliance (which is the opposite of impedance) is greatest when the air pressure in the canal is equal to that within the middle ear cavity; and it diminishes as the pressure increases or diminishes, thus causing the drumhead to be stretched. Different conditions in the middle ear produce characteristic changes in the graph thus obtained.

In the normal ear (Fig. 6.10, A), the graph is symmetrical, with a

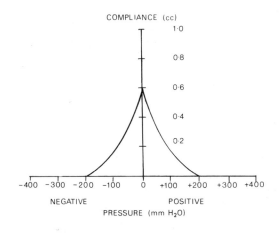

Fig. 6.10(A)   Tympanometry: Normal.

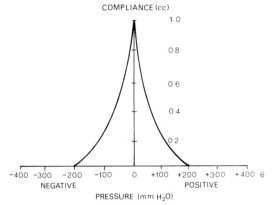

Fig. 6.10(B)   Tympanometry: Ossicular disconnexion.

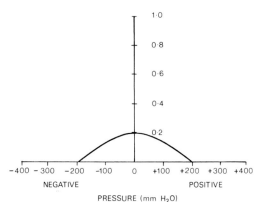

Fig. 6.10(C)   Tympanometry: Otosclerosis.

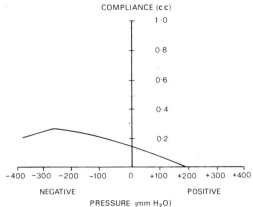

Fig. 6.10(D)   Tympanometry: Eustachian obstruction.

maximum compliance at 0 mm water and an average compliance range of approximately 0.6 cc; in ossicular disconnexion (Fig. 6.10, B), compliance is usually increased, and if a 800 Hz probe tone is used, there may be a double peak in the graph; when the ossicular chain is immobilized, as in otosclerotic fixation of the stapedial footplate, (Fig. 6.10, C), the middle ear pressure is normal but the compliance is greatly reduced; and when the Eustachian tube is blocked and the drumhead intact (Fig. 6.10, D,), the graph will show a negative pressure (of, for example, − 300 mm water) in the middle ear, and, especially when there is fluid in the middle ear cavity, there will also be a decrease in compliance, as shown by a flat curve.

Intra-tympanic muscle reflexes may be measured with the same equipment as that used in tympanometry, the stapedius (acoustic) reflex being usually elicited by an acoustic stimulus, the tensor tympani (non-acoustic) reflex by a jet of air directed across the cornea of the eye.

In eliciting the stapedius reflex, frequencies between 500 Hz and 4000 Hz are generally used, and sounds of more than 70 dB intensity will normally cause the stapedius muscles to contract bilaterally, the minimum intensity required to evoke the reflex being called the Acoustic Reflex Threshold (ART). In recruiting (usually sensory) perceptive deafness, the ART is often less than 70 dB above the subjective threshold; in non-recruiting (usually neural) perceptive deafness, the ART is usually greater than 70 dB above the subjective threshold, provided that the neural pathway is intact; and in conductive deafness, the reflex may be unobtainable as, for example, in gross fixation of the stapes in otosclerosis. When it is obtainable, the ART usually lies at 70–110 dB above the subjective threshold.

In eliciting the non-acoustic reflex, the puff of air against the cornea causes the tensor tympani muscles to contract bilaterally; and the measurement of this reflex is used to assess the integrity (or otherwise) of the neural pathways concerned.

Evoked response audiometry

Electrical responses are 'evoked' by acoustic stimulation, at every level of the auditory neural system from the hair-cells in the organ of Corti to the projection areas in the cortex of the brain, and the various forms of evoked response audiometry are dependent upon the recording and interpretation of these responses.

The tiny electrical events which occur, physiologically, in response to acoustic stimulation are normally swamped by background electrical activity, and it was not until the advent and development of computer technology that it become possible to use 'averaging' equipment which suppressed the background activity and enabled responses to acoustic stimuli to be summated.

Each of the responses evoked by acoustic stimulation differs from the others in the latency of the response, and generally speaking, the latency of each is a stable characteristic of that response. Each one yields a particular piece of information and suffers from its own particular limitations; and each supplements the others rather than competing with them (Fig. 6.11).

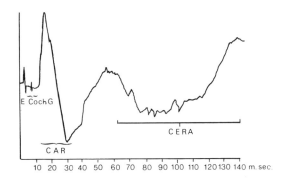

Fig. 6.11   Evoked response audiometry. This shows the latencies of the VIIIth nerve action potentials recorded by electro-cochleography (E coch G), the myogenic crossed acoustic response (CAR) and cortical evoked response audiometry (CERA). (After Douek, Gibson and Humphries).

In *cortical evoked response audiometry* (CERA), an averaging computer is used which, by 'time-locking' the responses in the cerebral cortex to acoustic stimuli, stores and summates these responses. At the end of a planned number (usually 40–60) of presentations of a pure tone of known frequency and intensity, at intervals of one-half to two seconds, a recording device attached to the computer gives a permanent record of the summated response. The latency of the cortical evoked response is a relatively long one, occurring from 30 to 130 milliseconds (thousandths of a second) after the onset of the stimulus. CERA is particularly useful in adults with non-organic hearing loss, functional overlay or malingering, and the thresholds produced by cortical evoked response audiometry in adults and older children are only 5 to 10 dB less sensitive than those produced by subjective pure-tone audiometry. Unfortunately, however, in children it is very often those in greatest need of assessment who are most difficult to test by this method, and sedation makes interpretation of the responses unreliable. It is not surprising, therefore, that otologists and audiological physicians have turned their attention to the other end of the auditory pathway, that is, to the cochlea itself.

In *electro cochleography* (E Coch G), the electrodes are placed in or near the ear to be tested. Two 'action potentials' are emitted, one by the cochlea itself (the cochlear microphonic), the other by the first neurone of the auditory nerve; but the cochlear microphonic potential is suppressed, by an artifice of subtraction, by means of an averaging computer, and it is the VIIIth nerve action potential which is actually recorded. The latency of this response is only 1 to 4 milliseconds. Some otologists use a very fine electrode which is placed on the promontory, either through an intact drumhead or through an existing perforation; and the stimulus generally used is a sharp acoustic click. Since the ear itself is mature at birth, electrocochleography can be used from the earliest days of life, but when the electrode is placed on the promontory, a near-threshold response can be recorded only from the basal turn of the cochlea, and thus it provides useful information only about the hearing for frequencies above 1500 Hz. Accuracy is within 15 dB, and the nearer the electrode is placed to the round window, the larger are the responses obtained.

In external electrocochleography, the electrodes are placed on the ear lobe or mastoid process and the top of the head, and some interesting waves are obtained; but since the responses are tiny, there is still considerable difficulty in using this type of test inclinical practice.

The *crossed acoustic responses* (CAR) are intermediate in latency between the nerve action potentials recorded by electrocochleography and the cerebral cortical responses recorded by cortical evoked response audiometry. They appear from 12 to 20 milliseconds after the stimulus, and they are evoked by electrical responses occasioned by contractions of the small muscles behind the ears. The active electrodes are simply pressed into position behind both ears, and the acoustic stimulus is provided either by clicks or by bursts of pure tones. Movements of the head may modify these 'myogenic' responses, by altering the muscle tone upon which they depend: for example, when the head is turned to one side or the other, the muscles on one side of the head and neck will relax, whilst those on the other side contract; hence, when an electrode is placed behind one ear only, the response may be completely abolished when the subject turns his head. It was for this reason that earlier attempts to make use of these responses were abandoned.

However, Ellis Douek and his colleagues at Guy's Hospital in London, realized that this response is a 'crossed' one, that is, that it can be recorded from both sides of the head, even when only one ear is stimulated acoustically, and they began to record the responses *simultaneously* from behind both ears, on separate channels of an averaging computer. When the response on one side of the head is damped down by head movement, it is often enhanced on the other side, with the result that a satisfactory response can be detected, down to near-threshold levels, on one or other channel, even in the most over-active child, and this without recourse to anaesthesia or even to sedation.

The crossed acoustic response also provides a quick, simple and painless test of brain-stem function.

These three main types of electric response audiometry are complementary one to another, each measuring the response to acoustic stimulation at a different level of the auditory pathway; and further developments in the future will, surely, open up a new era in which one day it should be possible to determine with reasonable accuracy the exact site of any lesion within the sensori-neural apparatus of hearing.

7. The Construction of Hearing Aids

The oldest aid to hearing is the hand cupped behind the ear, but this is of value only in the very slightest degrees of deafness. Non-electric hearing aids have been in use for at least two and a half centuries and they still find a limited usefulness in elderly persons who take unkindly to the mechanics of an electrical aid and cannot tolerate the distortions imposed on their hearing by the recruitment phenomenon (page 36). Ear trumpets, auricles and speaking tubes have all been used, but the best of these is the speaking tube which brings the speaker's voice acoustically nearer to the listener's ear. Undistorted gains of up to 20 dB may be obtained if the speaker will talk into the tube at a distance of not more than 2 or 3 inches from its speaking end.

The first commercial electric aid was made in America about eighty years ago, and great advances followed the invention of the thermionic (or radio) valve. There was a further rapid development in the design of miniature radio valves during the war of 1939–45 and these lent themselves to their incorporation in hearing aids. The substitution, in 1948, of the transistor for the radio valve led to a minor revolution in hearing aid design, and transistors are now used exclusively.

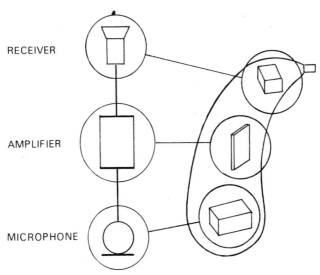

Fig. 7.1   The parts of a modern hearing aid.

Every electrical hearing aid consists essentially of three parts—a a microphone, an amplifier and a receiver (Fig. 7.1).

The microphone collects the sound energy and converts it into electrical impulses, which reproduce the rise and fall of pitch and intensity.

For a long time microphones were of the electro-magnetic type, but these gave a poor low frequency performance and the sound produced had an unpleasant, distorted quality. For a short time these were replaced by ceramic microphones which emphasized the lower tones and produced a more pleasant sound; but these were unstable and they have now been replaced, in the majority of modern commercial aids, by 'electret' microphones, which have the tonal qualities of ceramic microphones, with greater stability. (An 'electret' is a piece of material which is permanently electrically polarized, and the typical electret is an organic wax or plastic material of poor electrical conductivity).

'Directional' microphones, with front and rear sound entry, have recently been developed.

The amplifier may be an integrated circuit, consisting of twenty, thirty or even more components, including as many as nine transistors in a head-worn aid and up to twelve in a body-worn aid.

Printed circuits are in general use.

The receiver is of the insert type in body-worn aids; in the smaller head-worn aids it is placed inside the case of the hearing aid or in a spectacle frame. It receives the amplified electrical impulses and reconverts them to sound.

As with microphones, so with receivers, reduction in size can sometimes be achieved only at the expense of impaired technical performance, but for many body-worn aids, several types of receiver are available, with different frequency responses. Such a choice offers a wider selection of response curves and acoustic output power, and this permits a more satisfactory fitting of the most suitable instrument for each individual patient.

There are two main types—the air-conduction receiver and the bone-conduction receiver, the former being of the 'button' type, with a metal insert. The *ear mould* is an important part of the aid, and it is usually manufactured individually from casts of the external meatus. With ear-worn aids, the tube connecting the receiver to the ear mould acts as an acoustic filter, thus influencing the characteristics of signals, by cutting a part of the high-frequency range and adding new 'resonance peaks'.

There are, however, certain instances in which the use of an insert receiver is contra-indicated, especially when there is irritation, discharge or stenosis (narrowing) of the meatus; and it is in such conditions that one should consider the use of a bone-conduction receiver, even though its performance is usually inferior to that of an air-conduction receiver, save in a small minority of all hearing-aid users—probably not more than 2 per cent. The overall amplification in bone-conduction aids is limited to a small band of frequencies, and their battery consumption is greater. They are used with an oscillator and headband in body-worn aids, or built into the amplifier case in spectacle-type aids.

8. The Requirements of a Hearing Aid

'The requirements of an ideal aid are: high amplification, high fidelity, small size and weight, low power consumption and low cost. Objectives of low cost and light weight are directly opposed to the objectives of high fidelity, high amplification and long battery life.' Thus wrote Dr Fisch in 1954, and this was certainly true at the time his article was written. But since then the picture has changed radically and it is now possible, in the modern transistor aid, to combine lightness of weight with high fidelity, high amplification, and long battery life. Unfortunately, the cost of these aids (on the commercial market) remains high.

Amplification. It goes without saying that the first requirement of any efficient hearing aid is that it should make the sounds of speech loud enough to be heard by the deaf ear. The 'acoustic *gain*' (i.e. the difference in sound pressure level (in dB) between output and input) should never be less than 25 dB and some modern individual aids claim to provide a gain as high as 88 dB. Commonly, however, in order to avoid 'feedback', the gain is limited to about 55 dB in the middle range of frequencies.

The gain varies with frequency, and the relation between gain and frequency can be registered graphically as the *frequency-response curve* of a hearing aid.

Control of volume. The hearing aid user must be able to regulate the loudness of sounds coming through his aid, to meet the wide variety of situations and conditions in which he wants to use it. He needs a greater volume when he is listening to a speaker 10 feet away than he does when the speaker is only 3 feet away. This hand-operated volume control is present in every modern instrument and it allows also for the varying requirements of different users.

Limitation of output. Amplification must be distinguished from output, which is the maximum intensity that the aid can deliver. The maximum sound *output* of an aid is usually limited, deliberately, to about 120 dB sound pressure level (SPL); but instruments are available which are said to give 148 dB SPL. Overloading in this way produces 'harmonic distortion' of the sound output, and the wave-form then differs from that of the sound input. An aid with such a high output should be used with caution, and for limited periods, and especially in cases of sensori-neural hearing loss.

It is desirable, in certain instances, to limit the total output of a hearing aid—that is, to limit the total volume of sound delivered to the deaf ear.

Sounds which are excessively loud can cause discomfort and even pain. Discomfort is felt in the person with normal hearing when the sound intensity reaches a level of about 115 dB and this threshold of discomfort is reduced in persons with defective hearing. The more severe the hearing loss, the less tolerant is the deaf ear to loud sounds.

Sudden loud sounds are occurring, on and off, all day long—in the home, in the school, in the street, in the office and in the factory—the banging of doors, the opening and closing of desks, the explosive noises of traffic and machinery. Such sounds are distracting and uncomfortable and, if they are loud enough, there is even a possiblility that they may damage the hearing.

For this reason, some device is needed which will *automatically* limit the total output of a hearing aid, so that no sound will reach the deaf ear above the level of tolerance. Such a device is called Automatic Volume Control (AVC).

But there is more to it than this, for automatic volume control may also improve the intelligibility of speech, especially in cases of sensori-neural deafness. In the recruiting patient (page 36), the sensation of loudness increases with abnormal rapidity and he can therefore tolerate only a slight increase in the intensity of speech sounds. But sudden and rapid increases occur very often in speech, and the difference between the faintest and the loudest sounds in a single short sentence may be as great as 30 dB. When the sounds of low intensity (the consonants) reach him, he needs maximum amplification; as the intensity rises, he needs progressively less. Theoretically at least, an ideal form of automatic volume control would allow the faint consonant sounds to be amplified to the point of audibility without allowing them to be masked by the more powerful vowel sounds. In practice, this is not yet fully attainable, but such control should be incorporated in most aids which are to be worn by recruiting patients.

There are three methods of providing *automatic* volume control in a hearing aid—peak clipping, compression amplification and automatic gain control.

Peak clipping

In 'peak clipping', an electrical circuit is included in the amplifier system which ensures that the voltage fed from the output of the amplifier to the earpiece will never exceed a definite fixed maximum level which represents a safe limit of intensity for the deaf ear. Any increase in intensity above this level is 'clipped'; that is, it is simply not transmitted by the aid. The result (in terms of a single sine wave) is a distortion of the sound to a 'square' wave-form (Figure 8.1, A). Peak clipping therefore achieves its purpose at the expense of some distortion of the original sound wave. But the extent of this distortion

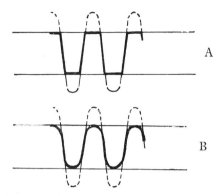

Fig. 8.1 Automatic volume control—effects upon the sine wave.
A, The effect of 'peak clipping'.
B, The effect of 'compression amplification'.

will depend on the extent to which the peak of the wave is clipped, and experiment has shown that the intelligibility of *speech* is unaffected unless the amount of clipping is very great, partly at least because the strong vowel sounds are clipped more than the weak consonant sounds.

Compression amplification
    The effect of compression amplification is to reduce the intensity of

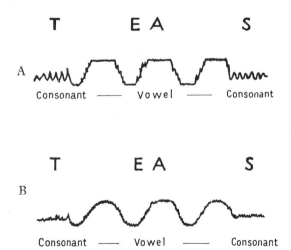

Fig. 8.2 Automatic volume control—effects upon the spoken word 'teas'.
A, The effect of 'peak clipping'.
B, The effect of 'compression amplification'.

excessively loud sounds whilst leaving the faintest sounds unmodified. The resulting sine wave has a pattern which is very similar to the original wave form (Figure 8.1, B). Automatic volume control is therefore achieved, by this method, with a minimum of distortion.

Whereas peak clipping is instantaneous, compression amplification takes a short but definite—only a very small fraction of a second—to come into operation. If we take the word TEAS (see Fig. 3.1), we can see the effect of these two methods of automatic volume control. Although the vowel sound 'ee' is rather distorted by peak clipping the consonants 't' and 's' retain their intensity (Fig. 8.2, A). Although the original wave-form is retained by compression amplification, and the intensity of the vowel sound 'ee' is reduced to a lesser extent than by peak clipping, the consonant sounds 't' and 's' are reduced at the same time (Fig. 8.2, B); and it is conceivable that this reduction of consonants (upon which the intelligibility of speech depends so much) may be a distinct *disadvantage* of compression amplification when we come to hearing for speech, as opposed to pure tones.

Automatic gain control

This form of control retains the crests of the waves and also reproduces their rising characteristic, but amplitude increases more slowly than with peak clipping or compression amplification. Control is exercised over practically the whole dynamic range of speech, and there is no perceptible time lag.

Peak clipping is easier and cheaper to incorporate in a hearing aid than compression amplification or automatic gain control, and it has been found to be preferred by many patients.

Adequate range of frequencies. It has been found experimentally that there is no loss of intelligibility of speech if frequencies below 500 Hz are cut out, and little or nothing is lost by cutting out the frequencies above 4000 Hz. The entire system of a hearing aid, including the microphone and the receiver, should therefore be capable of transmitting this range of frequencies and this requirement is achieved, more or less, in almost every modern aid.

Many variations are required and can be provided, the widest coverage available in any commercial aid at present being from 70 Hz to 7400 Hz.

Satisfactory frequency response. It has been suggested that the most satisfactory hearing aid for most patients would be one which was 'fitted' to his own particular pattern of hearing loss, in rather the same way as spectacles are prescribed specifically for each individual. In practice, however, this is neither practicable nor desirable, and most hearing aids today have a frequency response in which the high tones are amplified rather more than the low tones so as to prevent masking of the softer, high-pitched consonant sounds by the louder, low-pitched vowel sounds. It has been found, in fact, that the best frequency response is one in which there is a gradual increase in amplification from 300 Hz to 3000 or 4000 Hz at a uniform rate of about 7 dB per octave (J. J. Knight, 1967).

Modifications in the frequency response of a hearing aid can be effected in a variety of ways: by changes in receivers; by continuously adjustable tone controls; by varying the length and diameter of the tubing between the receiver and the ear mould, in head-worn aids; and by 'venting' of the ear mould. Vented moulds are claimed to cut down some of the background noise and to be useful in high-frequency hearing losses.

'Recoding' aids have recently been developed, notably in Denmark, by a process of 'frequency transposition'. Some deaf persons have a hearing loss which limits their residual hearing to frequencies below, say, 1500 Hz or even 1000 Hz. In such cases, a conventional hearing aid is of little or no value but, by filtering and modulating the high-frequency signals of incoming speech sounds to low frequencies, these 'transposed' signals are superimposed, on a 'signals amplifier', upon the low-frequency sounds transmitted through a conventional amplifier. Intensive auditory training is required before the wearer can learn to discriminate the distorted sound patterns thus produced.

9. Types of Electrical Hearing Aids

Most of our remarks so far have been concerned mainly with the individual hearing aid, though many of them can be equally applied to any type. It should therefore be appropriate, at this point, to describe the different types of hearing aid and to discuss some of the chief advantages and disadvantages of each.

Individual hearing aids. The greatest single advantage of the personal aid is that it can be worn throughout the waking hours without any

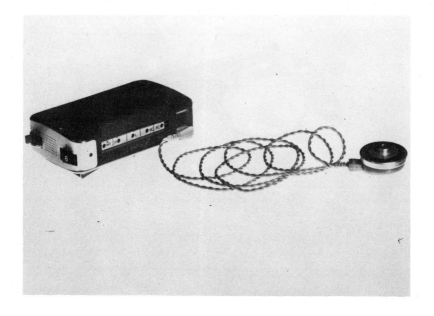

Fig. 9.1 Body-worn hearing aid, with air-conduction receiver attached. *(Kindly lent by R. Hawksley, Esq.)*

restriction of movement. The wearer if exposed to a constant atmosphere of sound.

There is now a very wide variety of individual aids and the vast majority of body-worn models are now of the 'monopack' type (Fig. 9.1) in which the microphone-amplifier units are both incorporated in a single case. The original National Health Service transistor hearing aid was of the monopack type and it was designed by members of the Medical Research Council and hence was known as the 'Medresco' (MEDical RESearch COuncil) aid (OL 56). More recently a behind-the-ear model has been introduced.

The first behind-the-ear hearing aid (known as the BE series) to be issued to adults on the National Health Service became available on 1st November, 1974. For the first year of this new issue, the instrument was available free of charge only to certain priority groups of users, including mothers with young children under 5 years of age; young people receiving full-time education: people receiving a war pension for deafness; and people with exceptional medical needs or some additional severe handicap, such as blindness. And it was estimated that a maximum of some 50 000 people in the United Kingdom would fall into the chosen categories.

Most, if not all, of these people have now been fitted with this aid, which is suitable for most persons who are moderately deaf; and one

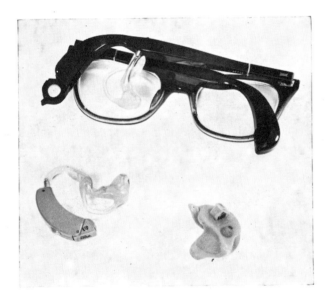

Fig. 9.2   Head-worn air-conduction hearing aids. *Top* – spectacle air-conduction aid; *bottom left* – behind-the-ear aid; *bottom right* – all-in-ear aid. *(Kindly lent by R. Hawksley, Esq.)*

year later, this aid became available to most deaf people of any age who are normally in full-time or part-time employment, and to those receiving full-time or part-time education.

This has been undoubtedly the greatest single advance in services for the deaf since the inception of the National Health Service in 1948 and, in addition to the new head-worn aids, there are also obtainable a number of high-powered body-worn hearing aids, by a special contract between the manufacturers and the Department of Health. Unfortunately, however, the supply of these more powerful instruments is limited to deaf children, and the deafened adult who needs a more powerful aid than those available through the Health Service must pay for his own.

In the commercial field attempts have been made, for several years, to make hearing aids smaller and smaller without loss of efficiency (Fig. 9.2). The most popular of these aids to-day is the post-aural ('behind-the-ear') aid, and there is now no difficulty in making batteries and electronic amplifiers small enough for these instruments; furthermore, the frequency response of the amplifier itself can be so designed as to make good some of the deficiencies of miniature microphones and earphones. Directional microphones are now tending to replace the backward—or downward-facing types in these models, with improvement in the wearer's ability to locate sound. The spectacle aid

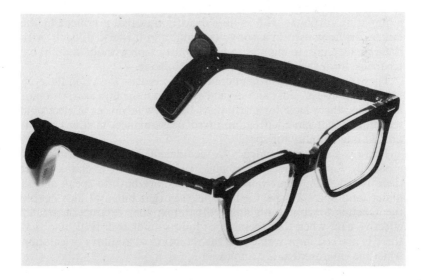

Fig. 9.3 Bone-conduction spectacle aid.

incorporates the whole of the 'works' within the limited space of a pair of spectacle frames and is particularly suitable for men. It is available also as a bone-conduction instrument (Fig. 9.3).

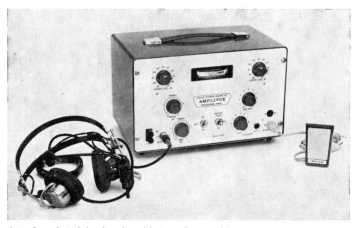

Fig. 9.4   Speech training hearing aid. *(Amplivox Ltd.)*
The teacher, or the child, can talk into the microphone *(right)*. Speech can be amplified, with very little distortion, up to very high intensity levels, and there is a separate volume control for each ear.

It is extremely difficult to produce small yet sensitive microphones and earphones which will give a smooth frequency response throughout the desired range; it is difficult to achieve a high sound output from a miniature earphone with as little distortion as that produced by the larger earphone used in a body-worn aid; and it is also difficult, with these smaller aids, to maintain a high acoustic gain without undesirable feedback from the earphone to the microphone.

These problems are further accentuated, needless to say, in the even smaller 'all-in-ear' aids; and in fact, apart from the miniaturization of amplifiers, there have for many years been few advances in electronic techniques that have led to improved performance, in terms of improved intelligibility for speech.

There is a growing tendency to recommend binaural hearing aids, especially for profoundly deaf children in whom it is claimed that there is a definite improvement in their ability both to speak and to understand speech. And Carhart believes that binaural aids enable them better to cope with noisy situations; that produce a greater effective gain when the reception of faint sounds is critical; and that there is marked improvement in the reception of auditory orientation when the environment is complex.

However, it must not be forgotten that the most powerful of modern hearing aids may possibly produce damage to the hearing through acoustic trauma. It is therefore essential to keep a very careful check on the hearing of such children with periodic audiometry, and one must be prepared to revert to a monaural aid if and when there is any sign of deterioration, at least until such time as it is reasonably certain whether or not that deterioration is due to the inherent nature of the deafness. All the same, it would be wrong to deny the optimal amplification of the most powerful aid available, at least to profoundly deaf small children, provided that this precaution is taken.

For binaural hearing, one may prescribe a single body-worn aid with a Y-lead; or two separate aids, either body-worn or head-worn.

The speech training aid. There are now available several makes of portable amplifier which can be used for auditory training and speech training in severely deaf children and adults.

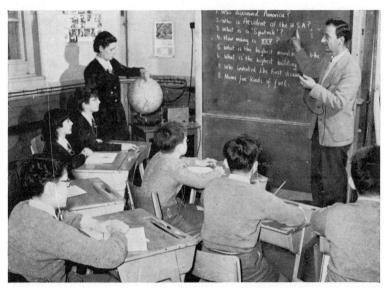

Fig. 9.5 'Loop induction' hearing aids in use at the residential school for Jewish deaf children, London. *(Multitone Electric Company Ltd.)*
The teacher speaks into his microphone and his voice is carried by a lead to the amplifier (on the small table, beneath the globe). The amplifier is connected to a 'magnetic loop', which encircles the classroom. Any child (wearing his or her own individual aid) can pick up the teacher's words through the 'induction coil' f the aid, in any part of a room so installed. For example, the girl pointing to the globe is still able to listen to her teacher, although she has moved away from her desk.

The speech training aid (Fig. 9.4) consists of a microphone, an amplifier (which incorporates a 'sound-level meter') and a receiver (usually carried on headphones, but alternatively connected with individual inserts). The speech trainer has a much wider frequency response than any individual aid, covering a continuous range of frequencies from 100 to 8000 Hz, and speech can be delivered to each ear separately over an intensity range of 85–135 dB, in steps of 5 dB.

The instrument provides speech reproduction of considerable clarity at very high intensities and it is capable of a much greater output, over a wide frequency range, than is normally available in the conventional individual aid. There is, therefore little distortion of speech.

The patient, whether child or adult, can listen not only to the speech of others but also to his own. In this way auditory training and speech correction are more effectively attained.

The radio hearing aid. Recently, radio hearing aids have been used in some special schools. They operate like an ordinary hearing aid but, instead of a magnetic induction coil, a radio microphone is used. The radio microphone transmitter is worn by the teacher, and the hearing aid also has an amplifier circuit—with volume and tone controls—and an output socket for the earpiece and lead. The child using such an aid is able to set the controls to suit his or her own particular requirements.

The induction loop aid. The induction loop system is used extensively in schools, especially in classes of younger children, to whom freedom of movement is so important (Figure 9.5). The child's own aid is fitted with an induction coil which picks up the sounds from a loop of wire which is laid round the walls of the classroom. The teacher speaks into a microphone which is connected to the amplifier system, and this in turn feeds sounds into the magnetic field provided by the loop of wire. Hence the sound is picked up by the induction coil of the child's aid and he is thereby enabled to hear at any part of a room so installed.

In this way a child's personal aid can be used at the turn of a switch, either as a class-room aid or as an individual aid, and this system has the added advantage that the quality of the sounds he hears, however little or however great their intensity, will be the same throughout the day.

This system can only be used with a body-worn aid.

The group aid. The group aid (Figure 9.6) is widely used in special schools. It consists of a teacher's microphone-and-amplifier control unit, and a pupil's control box with headphones. The amplifier has a frequency response of 30 to 20 000 Hz, and the pupil's control box has attenuators which deliver sounds from 0 to 135 dB SPL at the headphones. The apparatus allows for separate control of the frequency response for each ear, and thus enables the acoustic response for each pupil to be matched to his own particular hearing loss, thus providing greater intelligibility for speech. Since movement is severely restricted, the use of this equipment is confined to older children but, in common with the speech training aid, it possesses the great advantage of high amplification over a wide range of frequencies.

Other electronic aids to hearing. Many a hard-of-hearing person, especially the solitary housewife or the old-age pensioner, has little or no need to wear a hearing aid during the many hours spent alone; yet she may be often embarrassed by her inability to hear the ringing of a telephone or door bell. This applies particularly, perhaps, to the older

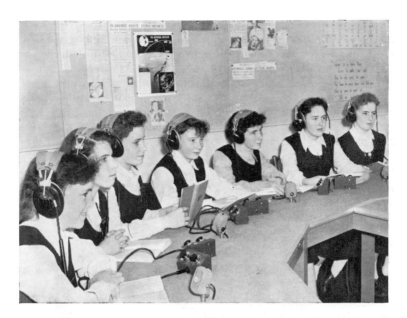

Fig. 9.6   Group hearing aid in use at the Royal School for the Deaf, Margate. *(Multitone Electric Company Ltd.)*
The teacher speaks into a desk microphone (not shown in the photograph) and his speech is fed from this into the amplifier. The volume controls and earphones are fixed attachments, and the use of the group aid is therefore limited to classes of rather older children.

person with a high-tone hearing loss, but it is not sufficiently well known that it is possible to have loud low-frequency bells fitted, either by the Post Office engineer or by the local electrician; and if a person has difficulty in hearing the telephone bell, an extension bell can be provided. There is quite a wide range from which to choose.

A handset containing a transistorised amplifier may be used instead of a normal telephone handset, with a volume control in the side of the earpiece; or an additional earpiece can be provided which enables a deaf perosn to listen to the incoming speech with both ears, and so reduce interference from other noises.

Alternatively, if a deaf person wears a body-worn hearing aid and wishes to use it with the telephone, he can place the earpiece of the telephone close to the microphone of the aid; if he wears a behind-the-ear aid, he may hold the telephone in the usual manner, adjusting the position of the telephone earpiece to obtain the clearest sound without whistling.

Any Area Telephone Manager will supply, on request, the leaflet DLE 550, which describes these various appliances.

Deafness may preclude a person so handicapped from listening to radio or television or records at a level which is acceptable to other members of his family or household, but there is now available a wide variety of adaptors. By plugging such an adaptor into the set, the hard-of-hearing listener is enabled to hear a programme through his own individual receiver, without disturbance to others.

The incidence of deafness amongst doctors is probably just as high as it is amongst their patients, and this may present difficulties in hearing the sounds of heart and lungs through a stethoscope. There are a few amplifying electronic stethoscopes on the market (Fig. 9.7), and one of the most recent models (Fig. 9.7) could be of great

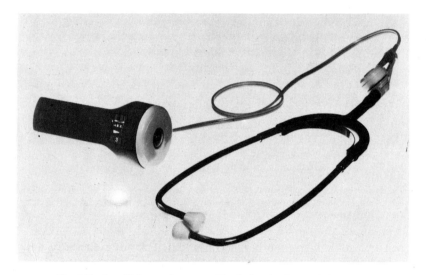

Fig. 9.7   Amplifying stethoscope. *(Kindly lent by R. Hawksley, Esq.)*

value both to hearing and to deaf doctors. This instrument not only amplifies the sounds, but transmits selectively those sounds which originate from the heart and lungs. For example, the 'first heart sound' has a mean frequency of 100 Hz, the 'second heart sound' one of about 120 Hz. Heart murmurs generally occupy the range between 600 and 800 Hz, and the highest pulmonary sound (as in 'bronchial breathing) has a frequency of just over 1000 Hz. The use of filters permits three different frequency adjustments to be made, and this instrument has a gain of over 40 dB.

10. The Choice and Use of an Individual Aid

The main function of a hearing aid is to make sounds louder but there are, of course, still cases of deafness in which an aid is of limited value, or none at all. This may be due to the extreme severity of the deafness, but much more commonly it is due to the type of deafness. And it will be remembered that it is in cases of sensorineural deafness that the 'recruitment phenomenon' (page 36) imposes a serious limitation on the usefulness of the aid. This is not to say that no case of sensorineural loss can benefit from one. Many thousands can and do. But it is a much simpler matter to help the patient with a pure conductive deafness, when the perceiving apparatus is healthy and the main problem is to make sounds loud enough to reach the normal cochlea at normal intensity.

There is available, through the National Health Service, quite a wide variety of hearing aids and, for children in particular, there is now practically no type of instrument that is not obtainable on the recommendation of an otologist. However, the range of aids available to adults is considerably more limited and, especially when a very powerful aid is required, those who can afford it tend to turn to the commercial world, where there is a wider selection of sizes, shapes and types—particularly in the field of head-worn aids, including those which are incorporated in a spectacle frame and are at present unobtainable at any age through the Health Service.

It is never an easy matter to advise on the choice of a commercial aid, for most manufacturers produce a wide range of models and there is no one make and no one model which suits *every* deaf person better than the rest. Nor can a fair trial be made in the consulting room—of the otologist, of the manufacturer, or of the vendor. I have long since lost count of the number of times I have been told by patients that they were tested, to their entire satisfaction, in the *quiet* consulting room of the otologist or the vendor, only to be bitterly disappointed when they went out into noisy street, or office, or home. Consulting rooms are always quiet, but the world outside is not. And it is not in the quiet everyday conversation of the drawing-room or lounge that most deaf people experience the greatest difficulty. It is usually noise and distance that make the handicap most noticeable, and it is only under these circumstances that any aid can be given a fair trial—in the office, at the board meeting, in the 'pub', in church or at the theatre. And it is for this reason that I now insist that all my deaf patients be allowed a trial for at least a week, under just those circumstances where the difficulty in hearing is greatest. The only exception to this rule should be the patient who has already tried an aid and found it to be entirely satisfactory but now seeks confirmation that this is a reliable model and that nothing further can be done to treat his deafness by medical or surgical means.

No aid can be expected to perform at its best without properly-fitting ear moulds, but no manufacturer or agent should be allowed to refuse a trial on request and a straightforward sale 'over the counter' should always be discouraged. There is nothing in law to prevent this practice, but for many years the Royal National Institute for the Deaf (RNID) has provided an advisory service in this respect, and the industry itself now has its own ethical code, formulated by the Hearing Aid Industry Association. There is also a Hearing Aid Council, which was set up by the passing of a Government Act in 1968.

Each aid has its own peculiar characteristics—of size, and shape, and colour, and performance—and it is nowhere truer to say that 'one man's meat is another man's poison.' It is very noticeable, too that once a deaf person has become accustomed to his own particular aid, a better one (as judged, for example, by the semi-objective method of speech audiometry) may seem poorer by comparison, until he has accustomed himself to the different characteristics of the new aid. It is not suggested that speech audiometry is either practicable or desirable in every case, because there are many subjective characteristics which may influence the purchaser in his choice—particularly those of weight, appearance and tonal quality—and the final 'proof of the pudding is in the eating'. But it may be of great value in case of severe sensorineural deafness, both in children and in adults, where only slight differences in the intelligibility of speech may be all-important.

The wearing of a conventional body-worn aid should present little difficulty to most women, and the instrument can be made quite invisible for the day-to-day activities of the fully-clothed average housewife, by minor adjustments to her *coiffure* and *couture;* and indeed, the same applies to-day to many young men! However, given the choice, most people prefer a 'behind-the-ear' model.

For men, the least conspicuous type is the spectacle aid.

For the deaf child, the aid should be as light as possible in weight and as free as possible from any hindrance to his normal activities. At the same time, of course, it must be sturdy.

A hearing aid is rarely advised in cases of unilateral deafness, but when there is a considerable difference between the hearing in the two ears and there is still much useful hearing in the better one, it may be wise to wear the aid in the worse ear. However, in most cases when an aid is desirable, and there is little difference between the ears it is customary to wear the aid in the better ear. Less amplification is needed and this, in turn, means less distortion and lower battery consumption.

In rather exceptional circumstances, one may recommend a CROS (Contralateral Routing of Signals) aid to patients with a unilateral hearing loss, for use particularly in those conditions (such as a formal dinner) in which much background noise makes the sufferer unaware of the fact that someone sitting on his deaf side is even speaking to him. In a CROS aid the microphone is situated on the poor side, and therefore picks up sounds from that side; but they are 'routed', through an open and not an occluding ear mould, to the good side; and since the ear mould on the good side is open, the hearing ear receives sound from both sides. In cases of binaural deafness, with unequal loss on the two sides, a Bi-CROS aid may prove to be useful. This has microphones on both sides but delivers all sounds to the better hearing ear. The circuitry of such aids may be concealed in a spectacle frame.

No electrical aid, however refined, can amplify selectively the sounds of speech. All sounds that come within its compass are made louder and the new user of a hearing aid is struck, and often dismayed, by the same realization that comes so dramatically to those who have had their hearing successfully restored by surgery—namely, that the world is a very noisy place. The worse the deafness, the more marked and distressing is the sensation of noise, and it is better to use an aid too early than too late. Many deaf people are loath to do this, partly because they feel that it publicizes their handicap, partly because they fear that it will make their hearing worse. Both ideas are fallacious. The handicap of deafness is much more evident than the presence of an aid, especially when it can be effectively concealed, and there is no evidence at all that the use of an aid will ever make the hearing worse— except, possibly, in cases of very severe sensorineural deafness where exceptionally high amplification is fed into one or other ear without the precaution of some output-limiting device (see page 65). The fact is that most deaf adults for whom an aid is prescribed are suffering from deafness which, by the very nature of the causative lesion, is progressive. And the feeling that the hearing has been made worse is further aggravated by the *sudden* return to a state of *relative* silence when the aid is turned off.

The new user of a hearing aid has difficulty in sorting out the sounds he wants to hear from those he does not want to hear. He has to rediscover the meanings of various sounds and learn that much of the background noise, at first so troublesome to many, is a part of the normal emotional life of hearing people. He must learn to recognize and accept the limitations of an aid and be willing to find, by experiment, how to gain the utmost from his instrument; and sometimes he may require the services of an expert in order to obtain the maximum benefit from it. It may never be possible for him to take part in group conversation, and he will be advised to sit or stand as near as possible to the person or persons he wants to hear. The futher away he goes, the more amplification will he need. And this will bring to him more of the unwanted background noise.

He will soon find that acoustic conditions are particularly difficult in public halls, in cinemas and theatres, where the effects of reverberation of sound tend to be very disturbing and to reduce the intelligibility of speech. Under these conditions, he should sit as near as possible to the centre of the hall, or theatre, because sound waves travel outwards from their source in a semicircle and the middle segment of the semicircle contains the maximum intensity. The deaf listener should therefore sit as near as possible to the front of the speaker, pointing the microphone of his aid (which is often strongly directional) at the speaker; and many of the newer head-worn aids make use of a directional microphone.

He will find it easier to hear clearly in rooms which have soft furnishings, curtains and carpets than in rooms with hard plaster walls and tiled floors with little furnishing. This is because the soft materials help to absorb sound and prevent echoes. In rooms where there is a considerable echo effect, such as tiled bathrooms and kitchen, sounds will appear hollow and booming.

The design and performance of hearing aids have improved enormously in the last quarter of a century, and to-day losses of up to 90 dB can be helped with a head-worn aid, up to 100 dB with a body-worn aid. As these instruments continue to improve, so there will be fewer and fewer deaf persons who cannot derive at least some benefit from their use.

11. Affections of the External Auditory Canal

Since the external auditory canal is a part of the conducting apparatus. anything which obstructs it will cause a conductive deafness (page 35), but occlusion must be more or less complete before deafness is noticed.

Wax is by far the commonest cause of obstruction in the external auditory canal and the deafness is often noticed suddenly. Ear wax is, of course, a normal secretion (from the ceruminous glands) but in many people it is so soft that it finds its own way out of the ear and is removed by the daily routine of toilet. In some, however, it is much harder and it then tends to collect in gradually increasing amounts until it occludes the canal completely. The reason for the sudden onset of the symptom of deafness is that the wax, which has usually been collecting over months or years, is 'hygroscopic'. That is to say, it absorbs water. And a plug of wax which has reached the stage of almost complete occlusion may suddenly swell up and block the canal completely when water enters the ear. Hence, there is not uncommonly a story that the deafness was suddenly noticed after washing or swimming.

Little is known about the why's and wherefore's of wax, despite a great deal of research into its formation and constitution. Some form a lot, some form little. In some it is soft, in others hard. Beyond this little is known with certainty, except that once wax has formed and caused deafness, it is likely to do so again, maybe only a few weeks or months later, maybe many years later. In some cases it tends to be mixed up with skin debris from the lining of the canal, to form a very hard plug, when the condition is known as *'keratosis obturans'*.

The deafness caused by wax is not usually very severe, as measured by the pure tone audiogram, and it may be so slight that the Rinne response (page 39) remains positive. (Expressed in terms of decibels, the Rinne response usually changes from positive to negative at a level of about 25 to 30 dB). But the sensation of deafness may be very marked, partly because it is so sudden in onset, and partly because it is usually accompanied by a sensation of discomfort or fullness in the affected ear. One therefore feels much deafer than the audiogram would suggest.

The external auditory canal may also be occluded by the introduction of *foreign bodies* or, much more commonly, by inflammation of the canal walls. Since the canal is lined throughout by skin, any inflammation of its walls *(otitis externa)* must be regarded as a dermatitis or eczema; and not uncommonly it is associated with skin conditions in the scalp or on other parts of the body. Irritation is its most prominent symptom, and this induces all too often the desire to scratch the ear. And it is this which so commonly introduces infection into the skin; hence the swelling which causes the deafness.

Atresia (or closure) of the canal may be complete or partial, congenital or acquired. In cases of congenital atresia, the child may be born with a solid plug of tissues in the affected ear or ears. This may be quite superficial or may extend right down to the position of the drumhead; in these latter cases it is commonly associated with other congenital malformations, of the middle ear cleft and ossicles. Acquired atresia may result from a chronic, long-standing otitis externa; from injuries to the canal walls by accident or operation; or from gradual occlusion of the depths of the canal by the ingrowth of small bony projections. These *'exostoses',* as they are called, tend to appear in a trefoil arrangement but they are, by themselves, rarely large enough to cause complete obstruction. On the other hand, they may narrow the canal very considerably and therefore allow deafness to occur much earlier when wax gets down into the narrowing gap. The cause of these exostoses is not known but they may be related in some way not yet determined to the temperature and humidity within the canal. They are thought to occur more commonly in swimmers and those few remaining stoics who take a daily ducking in a cold bath. One such case that I saw many years ago occurred in a young man who had been, some years earlier, the high-board diving champion of Australia. *New growths,* both benign and malignant, may occur but fortunately they are very rare in this situation.

The tympanic membrane (or drumhead) is the party-wall between the external auditory canal and the middle ear cavity, and perforation of the membrane is most commonly caused by infection within the cavity. The drumhead may, however, be ruptured by injury from without and it is therefore appropriate to consider these traumatic perforations at this point. They may be caused by the penetration of foreign bodies or by unskilled attempts to remove them; by syringeing of the ear or by inflation of the Eustachian tube, especially when the drumhead is thin or too much force is used; by fractures of the skull base, when the line of the fracture passes through the bony ring to which the membrane is attached—bleeding from the ear is a sign which should always be looked for in head injuries; or by a hand-slap or other form of sudden compression, as in rapid descent in non-pressurized aircraft. Blast injuries were not uncommon during the war and one still sees, almost every year, a few cases of traumatic rupture of the drumhead after Guy Fawkes' Day. Regrettably enough, one also sees the perforation which follows a 'cuffing', sometimes from a parent, sometimes (allegedly) from a teacher, and sometimes from a spouse.

12.   Affections of the Middle Ear Cleft

Injuries to the middle ear and ossicles
More than a hundred years ago Joseph Toynbee, in the last paper he
ever wrote, in 1866, reported that the long process of the incus could be
separated from the head of the stapes by a blow on the head, and he
called the condition 'disconnexion of the ossicles'. Such a lesion must
have been very rare in those days, but the steady growth of motorized

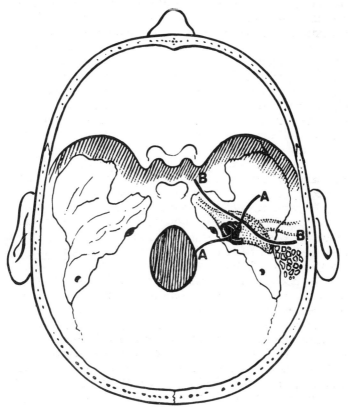

Fig. 12.1   Types of fracture of skull base.
A—A, Transverse fracture.
B—B, Longitudinal fracture.

transport has brought with it an increasing number of head injuries due to road traffic accidents; and many of the more severe of these injuries are associated with fractures of the skull base. When the temporal bone is affected, deafness may result; for this is the bone which contains the essential hearing structures.

Approximately three-quarters of all skull fractures involving the temporal bone are of the so-called *longitudinal* type (Fig. 12.1, B–B), and these are the fractures which may affect the middle ear and auditory ossicles. Bleeding into the middle ear (haemotympanum) or from the ear should always bring to mind the probability of a skull fracture, especially when it is accompanied by unconsciousness; but in most of these cases the hearing will return to normal within a few weeks. However, in a small proportion of them a conductive deafness, nearly always unilateral, persists after the tympanic membrane has healed and the haemotympanum absorbed; and in such instances, the otologist should suspect a traumatic lesion of one or more of the auditory ossicles.

These accidental injuries to the ossicles are not common, but the

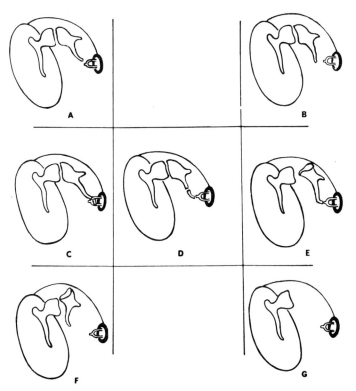

Fig. 12.2   Traumatic lesions of the incus (see text).

one most frequently affected is the *incus*. That this should be so is not surprising for, apart from a few strands of connective tissue, the incus lacks any form of anchorage by ligaments, whereas the *malleus* is attached, not only to the tympanic membrane but also (by a strong ligament) to the roof of the middle ear cavity, and to the anterior and posterior ligaments of the malleus; and the footplate of the *stapes* is fairly securely fixed in the oval window by an annular ligament.

Of all these rare but fascinating lesions, the commonest is a simple subluxation (Figure 12.2, A) or dislocation (Figure 12.2, B) of the incudo-stapedial joint; exceptionally, it may be impacted within the 'arch' of the stapes (Figure 12.2, C) or even fractured (Figure 12.2, D); and in some instances it has been found to be separated from the malleus alone (Figure 12.2, E) or from the malleus *and* the stapes (Figure 12.2, F); occasionally, the incus has been found to be missing altogether (Figure 12.2, G), and I have seen three such cases in which its absence resulted from surgical rather than accidental injury.

The crura of the stapes may be fractured (Figure 12.3, A), and sometimes its 'superstructure' (i.e., the head, neck and crura) may be widely separated from its footplate (Figure 12.3, B) ; in very rare cases the stapes has become separated from the incus and impacted into the

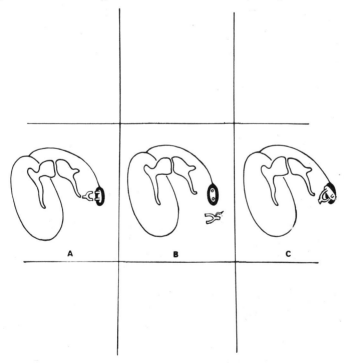

Fig. 12.3   Traumatic lesions of the stapes (see text).

oval window of the labyrinth (Figure 12.3, c). An added sensorineural deafness is usual in such instances.

Least commonly of all, the malleus may be torn away from its attachments to the incus and the drumhead (Figure 12.4, A), or fixed to the roof of the middle ear cavity by fibrous or bony attachments (Figure 12.4, B).

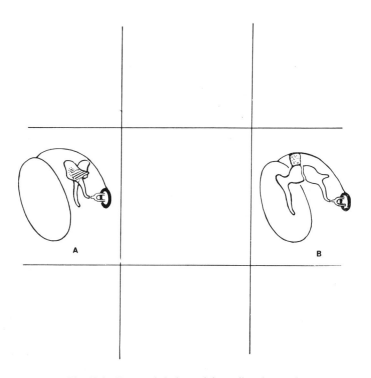

Fig. 12.4   Traumatic lesions of the malleus (see text).

Multiple or combined traumatic lesions of the ossicles may occur.

The diagnosis of these injuries depends upon the detection of a persistent conductive deafness following a head injury, after the drumhead has healed and blood has absorbed. Although the diagnosis may be established with near-certainty by acoustic impedance measurements, which show an increased compliance, its final confirmation depends upon the direct inspection of the middle ear through the binocular microscope, whose regular use in modern times has made possible their exact diagnosis and surgical correction.

It should be evident that all patients who have suffered from a severe head injury should be referred to the otologist.

Acute inflammation of the middle ear cleft

The whole of the middle ear cleft is lined by a continuous layer of mucous membrane, from the lower opening of the Eustachian tube to the furthermost cells in the tip of the mastoid process. This lining is continuous, at the tubal orifice, with the sheet of mucous membrane that lines the whole of the upper respiratory tract, and its ramifications into the nasal sinuses. The middle ear cleft should therefore be regarded as an integral part of the upper respiratory tract from which it develops.

Acute infections of the upper respiratory tract can spread very rapidly over the whole surface of the middle ear cleft and it is wise to assume that, once the cleft has been invaded, there is some degree of inflammatory change throughout its whole extent. On the other hand the process may be arrested at any stage, either by treatment or by Nature's defences.

By far the commonest cause of acute inflammations in the middle ear cleft is the common head cold, but any infection of the upper respiratory tract can spread to the cleft. Particularly does this apply to the acute upper respiratory infections which so often herald the onset of infectious fevers in childhood, especially measles and scarlet fever. These acute infections of the cleft occur most commonly in the years of early childhood, whatever their cause, and about three-quarters of them occur in the first ten years. It is not surprising, therefore, that they are very often associated with tonsillitis and adenoids.

The type of inflammatory reaction and its progress depend not only on the virulence of the infecting organisms and the age and resistance of the patient, but also on the treatment used and the stage at which it is instituted.

Anything which obstructs the Eustachian tube or interferes with its opening may also lead to inflammatory changes within the cleft. The tubes are normally opened by muscular action, and the acts of swallowing and yawning cause contraction of the muscles which clothe the tubes. This allows the air pressure within the middle ear cleft to be raised to that of the surrounding atmosphere, but if it cannot be opened the pressure within the cleft falls and the tympanic membrane is pushed inwards by the greater pressure of the atmosphere. This causes restriction in the movements of the membrane; the tube is 'locked' and deafness follows. Locking occurs when the difference in pressures between the cleft and the atmosphere is so great (usually at a difference of 80 millimetres of mercury) that it can no longer be overcome by muscular action, and the commonest causes are rapid descent in an aircraft, or compression in a diving-suit. These 'baro-traumatic' effects are more likely to occur in passengers who sleep in a plane (when the movements of swallowing and yawning are suspended or reduced) and those who fly with an upper respiratory infection. The sensation of locking must also be familiar to the many

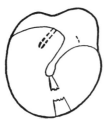

a. Broken light reflex

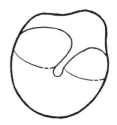

b. Fluid with 'hair line'

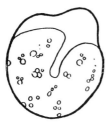

c. Fluid with bubbles

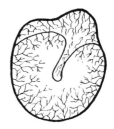

d. Injection of drumhead

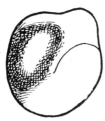

e. Bulging drumhead

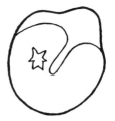

f. Recent perforation of
   drumhead

Fig. 12.5 Acute otitis media. Otoscopic appearances of the drumhead (tympanic membrane) in various stages of the infection.

thousands of people who travel by London's Underground trains between St John's Wood and Baker Street!

Tubal function may be impaired by malocclusion of the teeth, as in the syndrome described by Costen, or by restriction of the movements of the palate, as in the condition of cleft palate; and the tube may be invaded or squeezed by new growths in the nasopharynx (page 4). These rather rare tumours may present not uncommonly as cases of unilateral conductive deafness.

Occlusion of the Eustachian tube *(acute Eustachian salpingitis)* is the first pathological change to occur when the middle ear cleft is involved in an inflammatory process. A sensation of fullness is experienced in the affected ear and slight deafness follows. The tympanic membrane appears to be indrawn; the handle of the malleus looks foreshortened and its lateral process becomes more prominent. The surface of the drumhead loses some of its lustre and the light reflex may break up or disappear (Figure 12.5, a).

Engorgement and swelling of the cleft lining will follow if the process is not arrested, and exudation follows. As the exudation increases fluid collects in the middle ear cavity and sometimes in the mastoid air cells. The fluid is clear at first *(acute serous otitis media)* and the patient may feel a sensation of bubbling or fluid in the ear. The deafness is often noticed on rising from bed in the morning, as the fluid which has lain dormant in the air-cells over-night spills forwards again into the middle ear cavity. Occasionally the fluid may be seen through the tympanic membrane as a 'hair line' (Figure 12.5, b) and if the cavity is *filled* with fluid, bubbles of air may be seen (Figure 12.5, c). The drumhead will often look yellowish at this stage but tends to darken later; and if the inflammation is not controlled, pain ensues, the deafness progresses and the drumhead becomes red. At first the injection of the membrane is confined to the handle of the malleus and the periphery of the membrane (Figure 12.4, d), but later it becomes red all over and all landmarks are lost. The clear fluid changes to pus *(acute suppurative otitis media)* and the drumhead bulges (Figure 12.5, e). Finally, it bursts (Figure 12.5, f).

This whole chain of events may take place with astonishing rapidity and only a few hours may pass between invasion of the cleft and rupture of the membrane, especially in children. In a few cases of otitis media following measles or scarlet fever, the infection may be exceptionally severe and there is then a massive and sometimes painless destruction of the tympanic membrane *(necrotizing otitis media)*.

On the other hand, the inflammatory process may be arrested at any stage, either by Nature or by treatment, and it is expected nowadays that the vast majority of these infections will be controlled by one or the other, or both. At least it can be said today that no acute infection of the middle ear cleft can be regarded as cured until the tympanic membrane has healed and the hearing returned to normal.

If the drumhead fails to heal after 3 or 4 weeks, either after a single attack or after repeated attacks of acute otitis media, the patient may be left with a permanent perforation, when the condition is referred to as the 'safe' type of *chronic suppurative otitis media* (see below).

If the membrane heals but the hearing remains defective, one must always suspect that 'glue' has remained in the middle ear.

Chronic inflammations of the middle ear cleft

The 'Glue' ear

Otologists have become increasingly conscious, over the last decade or so, of the condition that has come to be known, almost universally, as the 'glue' ear. No doubt it has existed for much longer than is generally realized; and its more widespread recognition is no doubt due, at least in part, to the regular use in otological practice of the operating microscope. But there is equally little doubt that its incidence has grown enormously since the routine use of antibiotics in the treatment of acute otitis media. What happens, in essence, is this.

A child—for acute otitis media is mainly a disease of childhood—is sent home from school or wakes in the night, crying with earache. The doctor is called in by the parents—for nowadays this is almost exclusively a disease of General Practice—and he finds a red, sometimes bulging, drumhead. An antibiotic is prescribed, usually by mouth, and within a few hours or a day or two, the earache subsides and the child feels and looks better. Far too often the parents, relieved by the marked improvement, stop the drug too soon or give it too erratically, no longer stimulated to give the next dose by the earlier constant reminders of pain. Perhaps only one ear is affected, and in time the incident is forgotten—but only until, a few days or weeks later, the whole sequence recurs. The recurrence often takes place in the same ear; but in fact it is probably not a true recurrence but rather a recrudescence of an infection which has never really been fully controlled. Another course of antibiotics is prescribed and given, and again the condition appears to settle.

Sooner or later, with the passage of time, both ears will usually become affected; and it is not until both ears are affected that it dawns slowly on the consciousness of the parents or the teachers, that the child is not hearing properly. At this stage the advice of an otologist may be sought, and the child is found to be partially deaf. When he looks at the ears, the membranes are found to be intact but on one or both sides there will be some slight departure from the normal appearance of a healthy drumhead—a slight retraction, or an 'oily' appearance, or an amber-coloured tinge, or sometimes a dark plum colour. 'Glue' is diagnosed.

What, then, is this 'glue'?

The middle ear is lined by a mucous membrane containing mucous glands. When this membrane is inflamed, the mucus exudes in excess. If suppuration supervenes, mucus turns to muco-pus. The antibiotic controls the suppuration, and soon the muco-purulent fluid again becomes mucoid. But by this time, the Eustachian tube has become blocked, and in any event the mucus is now too thick to be evacuted spontaneously down the tube. And so it remains in the middle ear— and incidentally, forms an ideal 'culture medium' for future infection.

This mucus is the 'glue'. It is basically an active inflammatory exudate, and the condition is properly referred to as *exudative otitis media*. This is quite different from the passive transudation of clear watery fluid which is found in cases of simple mechanical blockage of the tube, due (for example) to the 'locking' of the tube caused by flying with a cold or the rare malignant tumours of the nasopharynx, and widely known as serous otitis media, or preferably *transudative otitis media*.

No one realizes more clearly than the present writer that this brief account is a gross over-simplification of a highly complex problem. It is almost certain that in the vast majority of cases of non-suppurative otitis media there is *some* exudation and *some* transudation. But the simplification is intentional; and it is intended merely to emphasize that in the one condition (exudative otitis media) the process of exudation is critical; whilst in the other (transudative otitis media), transudation is paramount. Be that as it may, there is no doubt at all in my own mind, after an extensive prospective survey, that the 'glue' ear is found most commonly, but not exclusively, in children who have had frequent attacks of acute otitis media treated with antibiotics.

What would happen if these children were not so treated? In some cases the simple uncomplicated infection in the middle ear would almost certainly become complicated by that acute infection of the mastoid which was the most feared sequel to acute otitis media before the late Sir Alexander Fleming's discovery of penicillin. Now, in its place, we have the 'glue' ear. So this is not a criticism of antibiotics, but we must regard the condition of exudative otitis media as the price we may have to pay, in some cases, for the virtual elimination of the once-dreaded 'mastoid'—not a heavy price to pay when we remember the alternative.

Chronic suppurative otitis media. It has been said earlier that a perforation may be left permanently in the tympanic membrane after single or repeated attacks of acute otitis media, especially when these are of the 'necrotizing' type which used commonly to complicate the infectious fevers of measles and scarlet fever. Occasionally a traumatic perforation may remain open.

The perforation in such cases is usually central and often large (Figure 12.6), and most of the time the ear is dry. However, every time the patient has a fresh upper respiratory infection, or alternatively when water is allowed to enter the ear, it will tend to discharge. But the infection is usually short-lived and soon the ear becomes dry again—until the next head cold or the next bathe. This cycle may be repeated time and time again, but the *discharge* is intermittent; it is mucoid and without odour; the ossicular chain is often intact; and there is no risk of serious complications. The condition is referred to as the *'safe'* type

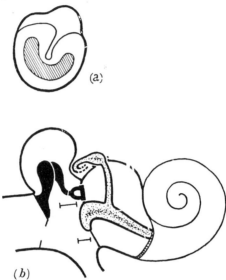

Fig. 12.6   Chronic suppurative otitis media—'safe' central perforation. (a) The perforation as seen through the otoscope (compare with Figure 2.4). (b) The effect of the perforation on hearing. The perforation is seen below the handle of the malleus. Sound energy at the oval window is slightly less than normal, that at the round window slightly greater (compare with Figure 4.2). The 'differential' between the two windows is therefore reduced, and deafness results.

of chronic suppurative otitis media, in which *the deafness* is often surprisingly slight, varying from 10 to 30 decibels. The sound energy transmitted to the oval window through the chain of ossicles is reduced but it remains greater than that at the round window (Figure 12.6, b) (see page 27).

Even if the membrane heals it may be left thickened and scarred, or adhesions may occur around the ossicles and labyrinthine windows, so producing the condition of *chronic adhesive otitis media,* with resultant deafness.

The *'dangerous'* type of infection is essentially different. It begins insidiously, and although it is seen more commonly in adults than in children, its origins are nearly always in infancy and early childhood, when adenoids and catarrhal infections of the upper respiratory tract are so common. These may give rise to a state of chronic obstruction of the Eustachian tube which results in defective aeration of the middle ear cleft, and also to 'frustration of pneumatisation' of the mastoid process which results in the 'ivory' type of mastoid so often associated with this type of infection.

Over the course of many months, or more commonly of many years, a negative pressure (or vacuum) is built up in the middle ear cavity, and one or other of the weaker areas of the drumhead (see page 8) is drawn in towards the cavity. All the time this is going on there occurs, *pari passu,* a slow and imperceptible disturbance in the normal migration of the keratin shed by the outer epithelial layer of the membrane (see page 4); and the keratin comes to fill up the deepening retraction pocket, most commonly in the attic. Eventually the weakened portion of the drumhead gives way, often silently and without the announcement of any symptoms, and the keratin enters the middle ear through the perforation so formed. In time, further layers of this 'skin' enter the cavity, to deposit themselves in successive coats around the central 'nucleus', like the layers of a peral. This 'pearl' is referred to conventionally as a *cholesteatoma.*

Once this process has begun it tends to advance, slowly but relentlessly, and sometimes comes to occupy the entire middle ear cleft, until such time as some complication or other threatens or supervenes, thus producing symptoms (sometimes for the first time) which bring

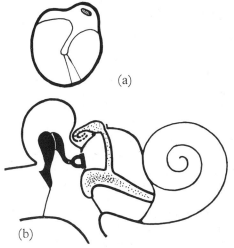

Fig. 12.7 Chronic suppurative otitis media—'dangerous attic perforation. (a) The perforation as seen through the otoscope. (b) Diagrammatic representation of the state of the ossicular chain. The deafness is only slight.

it to the attention of the patient and his medical advisers. For although a cholesteatoma is soft and putty-like in consistency, it has the ability to erode; and when this happens, complications (always severe and sometimes fatal) may occur. These include facial paralysis, meningitis and brain abscess; and, not least tragic in its consequences, invasion of the inner ear from the middle ear, with the subsequent conversion of a simple conductive deafness (sometimes severe but sometimes quite trivial) into a permanent irreversible sensori-neural deafness (often total). And it is precisely the tendency of this type of ear to produce these complications, combined with the silence of its pathological progression, that makes it so dangerous.

Occasionally the sudden onset of a grave complication may present the first clinical evidence of the presence of a cholesteatoma; more commonly a secondary infection in such an ear, perhaps initiated by a head cold or by the entrance of water into the ear, will produce a discharge. And *the discharge* tends to be purulent and foul-smelling

The perforation is usually in the attic (Figure 12.7, a) or in the postero-superior marginal area of the drumhead (Figure 12.8, a); in very advanced disease, it may be subtotal, with complete absence of the incus and most of the malleus (Figure 12.9, a)

The extent of *the deafness* depends not only on the site and size of the perforation, but also and mainly on the extent of damage to the

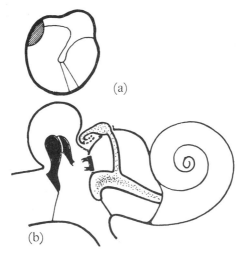

Fig. 12.8   Chronic suppurative otitis media—'dangerous' postero-superior marginal perforation. (a) The perforation as seen through the otoscope. (b) There is disruption of the ossicular chain between the incus and the stapes. Sound energy at the oval window is grossly reduced, that at the round window unchanged. The 'differential' between the two windows is markedly reduced, and severe deafness results.

ossicular chain. If the chain is intact, the hearing loss may be minimal, sometimes as little as 10 or 15 decibels (Figure 47, b); if there is a total loss of continuity between the incus and stapes (perhaps the commonest lesion), the deafness will be severe, usually between 50 and 60 decibels (Figure 12.8, b); when the drumhead has practically disappeared, and only the stapes or a part of it remains, the loss of hearing will be extreme, about 60 decibels or more (Figure 12.9, b). This last state is most often approximated when all diseased tissues have been removed by radical surgery.

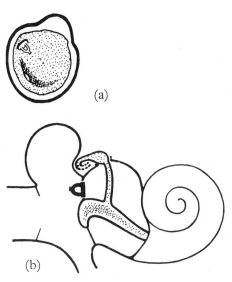

Fig. 12.9 Chronic suppurative otitis media—subtotal perforation. (a) The perforation as seen through the otoscope. The stapes is seen in the oval window. The round window niche is clearly seen beneath it. (b) There is complete loss of the malleus and incus, but the stapes remains mobile. Sound energy at the oval window is so reduced that it is almost the same as that at the round window. There is hardly any 'differential' between the two windows, and the deafness is very severe.

The above description of the 'safe' and 'dangerous' types of chronic suppurative otitis media gives no idea of the true complexity of the problem. To some extent the two types tend to overlap; discontinuity in the ossicular chain may occur in the so-called 'safe' type, and secondary infection may supervene at any stage in the natural history of the so-called 'dangerous' type. But this account has been intentionally simplified, to emphasize their essential differences.

New growths of the middle ear cleft

Growths rarely occur in the middle ear cleft but they are of slightly greater frequency than those in the external auditory canal. They may be benign (glomus jugulare tumour) or malignant (carcinoma), and deafness may be the presenting symptom with either of them. This is conductive at first, but may be perceptive later in both, if they spread to the labyrinth or auditory nerve.

13. Otosclerosis

'Otosclerosis' is a localized bony disease, and it means (literally) a hardening of the ear bone. But it will be remembered that most of the middle ear cleft and the whole of the inner ear are situated in the petrous portion of the temporal bone, which is one of the hardest bones in the the body (Peter = a rock). So this bone can scarcely become harder and the name is, in fact, a misnomer. Indeed the disease which has borne the name of 'otosclerosis' since Adam Politzer christened it thus in 1894 consists in a local replacement of the normal hard, mature

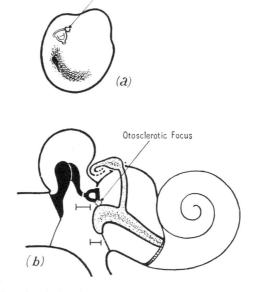

Fig. 13.1   Otosclerosis. (a) The 'otosclerotic focus' (drumhead removed). The disease is seen encroaching on the footplate of the stapes from the anterior margin of the oval window. (b) The effect of the disease on hearing. The sound energy at the oval window is reduced by the fixation of the stapes, that at the round window unchanged (compare with Figure 4.2). The 'differential' between the two windows is reduced, and deafness results.

bone with a soft, spongy immature bone; and the commonest site of origin of the disease is on the promontory, immediately in front of the oval window. This spongy bone—the French call the disease 'otospongiose'—spreads slowly, to involve and sometimes surround the margins of the oval window. More rarely the cochlea is also involved.

As the disease progresses, it encroaches upon the narrow area between the margins of the oval window and the footplate of the stapes (the vestibulo-stapedial joint); and it is its encroachment on the stapedial footplate which causes the deafness of otosclerosis. As the disease tends to progress, so does the deafness. As the footplate becomes more and more fixed, so does the amount of sound energy delivered to the oval window become further and further reduced and the 'differential' between the two windows diminished (Figure 13.1, a and b). The clinical picture then, is of a progressive deafness, conductive in nature, with a perfectly healthy middle ear cleft as far as can be seen by physical examination.

The deafness is most commonly noticed in the third decade; the patient is a young woman slightly more often than a young man; there is a similar deafness in some other member of the family in about half the cases; and not uncommonly it is first noticed, or greatly aggravated, by childbirth.

Both ears are usually affected and otosclerosis accounts for about half of all cases of bilateral conductive deafness seen in clinics. Many otosclerotics hear better in noisy surroundings— the *paracusis* of Willis (page 35)—as in a car, or a train, or a factory. The voice is often soft and flat.

No one knows the cause of otosclerosis though several theories have been advanced. Its association with pregnancy has suggested a possible hormonal origin, and its tendency to occur in families bespeaks an inheritance as the causative factor. It is also thought by some that the disease process is accelerated by repeated upper respiratory infections, and several studies in twins have shown that the deafness tends to be more advanced in the one who has been subjected more frequently to colds. But the cause remains uncertain.

There are certain generalized bony diseases which tend occasionally to localize in this important part of the skeleton, and the one which most closely resembles otosclerosis is the condition of Fragilitas Ossium. As its name implies, the bones are fragile and they fracture easily. The condition tends to occur in families and the sufferers are further distinguished by blue sclerotics—the 'whites' of the eyes are blue. Deafness may also occur and it resembles otosclerotic deafness very closely; indeed, it may be indistinguishable from otosclerosis. The combination of fragile bones, blue 'whites' and otosclerotic deafness is known as the van der Hoeve-de Kleyn triad.

Deafness is a frequent symptom in cases of Paget's disease (osteitis deformans), a condition in which the skull bones tend to be enormously thickened. (It is sometimes first noticed by the patient because he has to take a larger size in hats.) The deafness may be conductive or perceptive; in the former instance, it is possibly due to deposition of calcium in the vestibulo-stapedial joint.

Conductive deafness may be caused by the so-called 'eosinophil granuloma', which is characterized by localized bony lesions in its early stages, sometimes of one bone, often of the temporal bone. X-rays may show massive destruction of its petrous portion. Discharge may also occur, and the condition may simulate a chronic infection.

14. The Conservative Treatment of Conductive Deafness

Re-opening closed channels

Conductive deafness is often referred to as obstructive deafness. It may be caused by anything that obstructs the external canal; it may be caused by anything that obstructs the Eustachian tube; and it may be caused by anything that obstructs the movements of the drumhead or ossicles. And removal of the obstruction will often cure or relieve the deafness.

Removal of obstructions in the external auditory canal. It is usually a fairly simple matter to remove wax either with a probe or by syringeing, but it may be extremely difficult to remove it when it becomes impacted with a mass of skin (keratosis obturans). A general anaesthetic may sometimes be necessary in such cases.

Foreign bodies may also be extracted by syringeing, especially when they are small in size and irregular in shape. Special care is needed, however, in removing a smooth, rounded foreign body, especially when it causes complete obstruction.

Otitis externa will usually yield readily to simple conservative treatment, but it must never be forgotten that this is a skin condition, that the skin may be sensitive to antibiotic drugs, and that their local application may cause more swelling, more obstruction, more discomfort and more deafness. Bland applications will reduce the swellings of the walls, and one sees some strikingly successful results from the local application of cortisone preparations, even in chronic cases of long standing. It is in these cases, however, that the swelling may be marked and resistant, with permanent obstruction from the swelling of the skin. In such cases, as in the narrowing (atresia) which sometimes follows a direct injury to the canal, the opening may be gradually enlarged by the insertion of polythene or rubber tubes in successively larger sizes; rarely, surgery may be necessary.

All of these conditions can and should be cured with simple conservative treatment, and restoration of normal hearing should be the rule.

Unblocking the Eustachian tube. The Eustachian tube may be blocked, as any other tube, by something within its lumen; by swelling of its walls; or by anything that presses on it from without. Most commonly, it is blocked by an inflammatory process (salpingitis); less commonly, by pressure changes (barotrauma); rarely, by growths. Not uncommonly a tube which is blocked by swelling can be opened by the use of simple decongestant drugs, usually by mouth; but when the blockage is resistant to such simple treatment, it can often be relieved, if only for a short time, by blowing air up it.

Inflation of the tube

Many people experience a sensation of crackling or popping in their ears when they blow their noses forcibly at the height of a cold. They have blown air up a blocked tube.

It is not suggested that air *should* be blown up the Eustachian tube at the height of a cold. On the contrary, it may easily introduce infected secretions into a middle ear cleft that is already vulnerable. But the patient may afford himself considerable relief to a 'dry' blockage if he blows out forcibly whilst holding his nose and closing his mouth. This manoeuvre was first rationalized by Antonio Valsalva, who lived in the late seventeenth and early eighteenth centuries, and it may be recommended to those who feel their ears blocking when they fly—unless, of course, they have a cold, when they should not be flying anyway. It has, however, one obvious disadvantage—that it acts more forcibly on the normal ear when only one is affected.

Another disadvantage, perhaps less obvious, is that many people find it quite impossible to do it; and for such persons Politzerization may be tried. This method of inflation was first described by Adam Politzer of Vienna, who died in the early part of the present century.

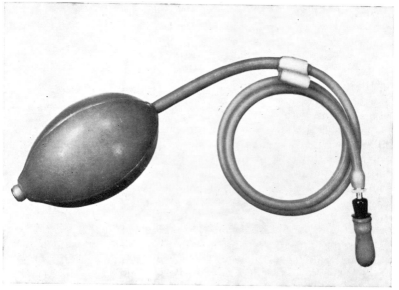

Fig. 14.1   Politzer bag, with soft rubber nozzle. (*Down Bros. and Mayer and Phelps.*)

A soft rubber nozzle is attached to a Politzer bag (Figure 14.1). The patient is asked to take a sip of water and hold it in his mouth. The nozzle is inserted into one nostril, the other being closed by the otologist's finger, and when all is ready, the patient is instructed to swallow. As he swallows, the palate rises and closes the mouth off from the nasopharynx; the 'Adam's apple' (part of the larynx) rises; and as it rises, the bag is compressed. The air is unable to escape into the nose, because it is closed off by the nozzle and a finger; it cannot escape into the mouth (unless the palate is cleft) because the palate rises as we swallow; it can only go up the tubes and into the ears—theoretically, at least. But it does not always work that way, and it is open to much the same objection as the Valsalva manoeuvre when the blockage is confined to one tube. Nevertheless, it can be very useful in children.

The most certain way of inflating a blocked tube—but not the easiest and not the most comfortable—is by catheter. The Eustachian catheter (Figure 14.2) has a gently curved beak which can be advanced along the floor of the nose and turned outwards until its point comes

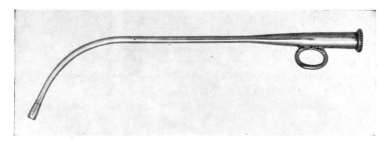

Fig. 14.2   Eustachian catheter. *(Down Bros. and Mayer and Phelps.)*

to occupy the lower opening of the tube. The other end of the catheter is attached to the Politzer bag, which is squeezed. By this method, air can be made to enter each tube separately and the otologist can confirm that air has entered the tube (or not) by attaching his own ear to the patient's through the medium of an auscultation (or listening) tube, usually referred to as Toynbee's otoscope.

Removal of surrounding obstructions

Removal of adenoids (and tonsils)

Apart from the transient tubal blockage which so commonly follows an acute infection of the upper respiratory tract, there are several conditions which may cause a more permanent obstruction; these include malocclusion of the teeth, which can be corrected by prosthetic treatment. But by far the commonest is adenoids; and tubal dysfunction may also result from gross enlargement of the tonsils, especially at their upper 'poles'. It is therefore not surprising that *removal of the adenoids,* and sometimes also of the tonsils, is widely advocated as the first line of treatment in those thousands of children who suffer from repeated attacks of Eustachian obstruction with each and every head cold.

There can be no doubt that many children are better for this relatively minor procedure. It does not prevent further colds which are, after all, the main cause of the trouble. But the subsequent effects of these colds tend to be less serious, and the bouts of Eustachian salpingitis tend to be less frequent, and shorter-lasting when they do occur.

On the other hand, one sees many children in whom the attacks of salpingitis—and, often, of otitis media—have actually dated from the operation, and others in whom the attacks appear to have been worse. It is certainly not the whole answer to the problem. If it were, there would be no other treatment; but several other forms of treatment have been advocated by some authorities, including radiotherapy.

Irradiation of the nasopharynx

There is no denying the value of radiotherapy in the treatment of malignant new growths in the nasopharyns and it is fortunate that they tend to be highly sensitive to radiation. One has seen them almost literally melt away under the influence of radiation, with rapid relief of the deafness, often within a few days. And there was a vogue, some fifteen to twenty years ago, for treating 'benign hyperplasia' of the lymphoid tissue in the nasopharynx by irradiation.

It was Samuel Crowe, in the United States, who popularized this form of treatment. We know that the tonsils and the adenoids are not the only collections of lymphoid tissue that can become enlarged and inflamed, for this type of tissue can also occur around the openings of the tubes, and it has also been thought (on very flimsy evidence) to occur within the tubes themselves. So, it was argued, if these attacks of salpingitis recurred after the tonsils and adenoids had been removed, the treatment should be directed to those collections of lymphoid tissue which occurred in and around the tubes. And lymphoid tissue, said Crowe, was sensitive to *irradiation.* Hence a new method of treatment was devised, whereby these areas were irradiated either by radium applied locally to the openings of the tubes in the nasopharynx, or by external irradiation applied to the tubes from outside.

Some very impressive results were published, but no 'controls' were used. And it was perhaps not sufficiently realized that this condition of recurrent Eustachian salpingitis was one of the few of which we could say, with complete confidence, that most of the children who suffered from it would grow out of it spontaneously, usually between the ages of eight and eleven. Those who did not were almost certainly suffering from what we now recognise as the 'glue' ear.

Following the publication of several controlled trials, the method has now been abandoned. Long-term results of treatment by irradiation showed no improvement over the natural spontaneous remissions that occurred in children not so treated; nor was it without its dangers. Children are particularly sensitive to the effects of irradiation, and therapeutic radiotherapy in children should be reserved solely for those tragic few who have malignant conditions.

Treatment of infections

Antibiotics. The treatment of infections has been radically influenced by the discovery of the sulpha drugs and antibiotics. It so happens that the vast majority of all cases of acute suppurative otitis media are due to infection with a limited number of organisms—most commonly the streptococcus, pneumococcus and staphylococcus—and that all of these organisms are (in the main) remarkably sensitive to penicillin.

Before the days of chemotherapy, the otologist's chief concern with these infections was to preserve life, for they could be extremely virulent and not without danger. Acute infections of the mastoid are now a rarity; but whatever the stage of the infection, nearly every case of acute otitis media today can be expected to clear within a few days, and the hearing restored to normal within three or four weeks.

There are, however, some cases in which deafness persists, and in some cases this can be relieved by inflating the tubes. But still there are a number of cases in which the deafness resists treatment, or recurs quickly and often. Rarely—in childhood, at least—this may be due to adhesions, but more often it is due to repeated reinfection of the middle ear cleft, commonly by repeated head colds. This may lead to the condition of 'glue' ear (see Chapter 12), and the treatment becomes surgical (see Chapter 15).

Removal of tonsils and adenoids—again! Constantly recurring infections of the upper respiratory tract constitute one of our biggest problems, and many hospital clinics are cluttered up with catarrhal children. The solution in some cases may lie in attention to a source of chronic infection in the nose, the nasal sinuses, the tonsils or the adenoids. Not uncommonly it is the tonsils and adenoids which receive our first attention, and there are certainly some children who appear to be much better after the operation. But some remain the same, others get worse, and it must be remembered that, as in recurrent bouts of Eustachian salpingitis, so in these recurrent attacks of otitis media, the middle ear cleft is merely sharing in a widespread infection of the upper respiratory tract (to which the cleft rightly belongs), and that there is a certain peak incidence (as in the common cold) in children of early school years. We must not forget that most children will grow out of these attacks between the ages of about eight and eleven, and we must be careful not to attribute the successes of Nature to the skill of the surgeon.

This was emphasized in a report made by a working party of the Medical Research Council and published in the *Lancet* in September 1957. Their survey was carried out by 28 general practitioners (99 per cent of all cases of otitis media are treated in general practice and never reach the hospital clinics) in 13 practices. Between them these doctors had over 47 000 patients, and during the year 1955 they saw 1162 patients with acute otitis media; 127 of them had had more than one attack during the year, and almost half of them had had previous attacks before the survey began.

'The disease,' says the report, 'is mainly one of the early childhood years—75 per cent of our cases were in children under 10 years of age—and tends to recur, the incidence diminishing steadily with age.'

'This age distribution is important in the correct management of the patients. A definite peak incidence was present in our cases at 3–6 years of age, this peak being followed by a dramatic fall in incidence in each subsequent year. This pattern has also been noticed by Fry (1957) in children with the common upper respiratory infections and in the more specific conditions of acute tonsillitis and acute chest infections. These findings suggest that the whole respiratory tract should be viewed as a single and continuous unit liable to similar natural changes. Any explanation of these patterns must at this stage be rather speculative, but they may be related to cross-infection by children mixing more in the pre-school and early school years, and they may also be related to physiological changes in children's respiratory tracts at the age-period 3–6 years. Whatever the true reason, this natural peak in the incidence of acute otitis media at 3–6 years and the subsequent fall must be clearly appreciated when considering radical therapy such as removal of tonsils and adenoids.' (This is of course surgical treatment, if not very radical surgery. But it is included in the present chapter on 'Conservative Treatment' to distinguish it from those surgical procedures on the ear itself which are designed primarily to restore or preserve hearing rather than to remove infection.)

'*Such data as were obtained,*' the report continues, '*regarding the significance of tonsillectomy and adenoidectomy in relation to recurrence of otitis media showed no difference that could be attributed to the operation.*'

This then is not the whole answer.

'Artificial eardrums'

The drumhead may be ruptured by injury, usually from without; or by infection, always from within.

In cases of traumatic rupture there is one vitally important principle of treatment which can be summed up in a phrase—*masterly inactivity*—inactivity because nothing active should be done; masterly because there is always a great temptation to want to do something. And it often requires much more experience and self-discipline to leave these things alone than to act. There is often some bleeding round the edges of these perforations, and any attempt to remove the protective clot is likely to introduce a secondary infection into the middle ear, with subsequent otitis media. When this happens, it can usually be controlled by antibiotics, but it should happen very rarely. In most instances a traumatic rupture will hear rapidly and completely, provided it is left alone.

There are, however, many thousands of people in Britain who carry with them throughout life an open perforation of one drumhead or both, sometimes a legacy of childhood fevers, rarely the price of a cuffing. They are often perfectly safe, central perforations. Sometimes they discharge with every fresh cold or with every swim; sometimes they have been dry for very many years; sometimes they have started so long ago that the patient may even be unaware that he has a perforation and he may resist, sometimes quite vehemently, any suggestion that he must have had trouble in the past.

These perforations may heal quite spontaneously after many years, and they may sometimes close after application of a caustic solution to their edges. This freshens the edges of the perforations, and appears to rejuvenate the process of healing. 'In some cases, with a dry median perforation,' to quote Scott Stevenson, 'the hearing may be distinctly improved by the insertion of a small cylinder of cotton-wool, moistened in liquid paraffin or sterile water, just touching the promontory through the perforation—finding the exact spot may require some manipulation. This method was invented so long ago as 1848 by Dr James Yearsley, and termed by him the "artificial eardrum". Other 'artificial eardrums' can also be placed over the perforation in the form of paper or plastic prostheses.

Aids to hearing

It will be realized that many cases of conductive deafness are amenable to treatment by simple conservative measures, and that cure is sometimes to be expected. There are also many other cases in which the hearing can be greatly improved by surgery. These include atresias, congenital or acquired; chronic infections of the middle ear cleft, active or quiescent; and otosclerosis. But even if treatment is unsuccessful or declined, the patient with a pure conductive deafness can always fall back on a hearing aid. If his deafness is purely a conductive one, it can be assumed that his neural apparatus is healthy. And if this is so, his one main requirement is that sounds shall be delivered to his normal cochlea at their normal intensity. In the vast majority of cases, this can be achieved satisfactorily with a good hearing aid (see Speech Audiometry, page 53). Sometimes, however, for reasons often unexplained he may have difficulty in understanding speech even through the best of aids and it may help him enormously to learn to lip-read.

Aids to seeing

When a child is born partially deaf, he will often learn to lip-read quite spontaneously. Many who are born totally deaf can be taught to lip-read, and one has only to see a few 'orally' successful deaf children to realize how valuable these visual clues to speech can be.

It is not suggested that the child or adult who acquires a profound deafness after he has learned to speak can ever master this elusive art with the same certainly as the infant, but we tend perhaps to underestimate its potential value for these older patients. As Scott Stevenson has written: 'It is only within comparatively recent years that lip-reading has been recognized as an aid to the adult deaf as well as a method of educating those born deaf. Lip-reading is by far the best single aid to the deaf adult; it never gets lost or out of order, and requires no repairs or batteries. As an adjunct to an efficient hearing aid, lip-reading plays a most important part in the rehabilitation of the deafened....'

15. The Surgery of Conductive Deafness

The surgery of serous otitis and the 'glue' ear

Serous otitis may occur as but a stage in the natural history of acute otitis media; and if the infection is controlled at that stage, either by Nature or by treatment, the patient (more commonly an adult) will have some deafness. The condition may also occur as a simple passive 'transudation', due to negative pressure in the middle ear, in blockage of the Eustachian tube caused (for example) by flying, or by new growths in the nasopharynx in the vicinity of the tubal orifice.

In any event the fluid will be thin and watery; and it may occupy the whole or only a part of the middle ear cleft.

In the type which follows a simple upper respiratory infection, the eventual resolution of that infection will usually be followed, sooner or later and usually within two or three weeks, by spontaneous opening of the tube and evacuation down it of the fluid. Hence it may clear naturally.

Failing this, the tube may be opened, either by politzerization or by catheterization, with the same result. When catheterization also fails to clear the fluid, it may be possible to introduce a small soft Weber-Lyall catheter through the metal Eustachian catheter and to clear the fluid by suction. If this too fails, resort must be made to the minor surgical procedure of myringotomy—an incision in the tympanic membrane.

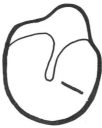

Fig. 15.1   Myringotomy.

Myringotomy. It is customary nowadays to perform myringotomy through the binocular operating microscope. A small radial incision (Figure 15.1) is made in the drumhead low down and far forward (in approximately the 5 o'clock position in the right ear, 7 o'clock in the left), so that it will be as near as possible to the upper opening of the

Eustachian tube into the middle ear.

When the fluid is thin and serous, simple myringotomy will usually provide drainage until such time as fresh fluid is being no longer re-formed—unless, of course, it is associated with permanent tubal obstruction as in a growth of the nasopharynx.

It is of the utmost importance that attention should be paid to the state of the upper respiratory tract, and every attempt must be made to reduce any co-existent congestion therein before any surgical attack is directed towards the ear itself.

The same applies to the 'glue' ear, found much more commonly in children. In these young patients the tubal obstruction may be caused or aggravated by enlarged adenoids and sometimes also by enlarged and infected tonsils. Indications of the removal of these obstructing agents must, of course, be considered on their own merits, but the surgical problems of the 'glue' ear are much more difficult than those of simple serous otitis.

The 'grommet'. Simple myringotomy is useless in true exudative otitis media, for the mucus is far too thick to escape through the incision. At the very least, suction is required. But even this is not enough, for the Eustachian tube is still blocked, the incision heals within a few days, and the inflamed lining of the middle ear continues to exude the thick 'glue'.

In these cases, therefore, an attempt must be made to create a 'controlled perforation'—something which will keep open the perforation for as long as it is required, not so much to let out fluid (for this has been removed by suction already and it is far too thick, anyway, to escape naturally) but rather to let air in (that is, to ventilate the middle ear deprived of ventilation by virtue of a chronically obstructed tube).

The most satisfactory way, to date, to achieve this controlled perforation is to insert through the myringotomy some form of tube which

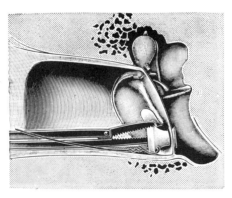

Fig. 15.2   The Shepard grommet. *(By courtesy of Messrs Down Bros. and Mayer and and Phelps. Ltd.)*

will remain in position for an adequate period of time; which is hollowed out through its centre to allow air in; and which is not so long that it becomes easily obstructed by wax. At the same time, it must be readily removable. The tube now commonly used for this purpose is the Shepard 'grommet' (Figure 15.2) a small plastic tube made of Teflon, with a dumb-bell constriction near the middle to hold it in position when the drumhead heals.

More and more otologists are tending to leave in these grommets for longer and longer, and there are even those who advocate their retention until adolescence. But herein lies one of the problems; for often they reject themselves spontaneously after a few weeks or months, after which it may be necessary to repeat the operation if the 'glue' reforms. In the average case, the grommet will be rejected after about 6 months, but occasionally it is retained for as long as 2 years, or even longer.

The grommet is by no means the whole answer to the 'glue' ear, and many problems still remain unsolved; but it is by far the most satisfactory method so far devised for the treatment of this often refractory condition.

It has been suggested that the 'glue' may be liquefied (and hence discharged naturally down the Eustachian tube) by the injection through the intact drumhead of certain chemical substances, notably urea; but a recent careful comparison of this method with insertion of grommets has shown the latter to be infinitely superior in the long term.

One of the many problems of the grommet is that in the opinion of many otologists, it precludes swimming. But this is surely a small price to pay for (in most instances) an immediate and permanent restoration of normal hearing.

The surgery of otosclerosis

Not every sufferer from otosclerosis is suitable for surgery, as the disease is by nature progressive and it tends, in time, to involve the cochlea. The various operations designed for the relief of otosclerotic deafness are purely mechanical, designed to restore the conducting apparatus as nearly as possible to a normally functioning state. They cannot possibly improve any hearing loss due to cochlear involvement.

The state of the cochlea can be roughly assessed by the patient's ability to hear by bone conduction (page 42). Usually it is remarkably good in otosclerotics, except in the most advanced cases or in those rare cases which tend to affect the cochlea first and sometimes alone. The audiometric measurement, of hearing by bone conduction is therefore always advisable in the selection of cases for operation. Success is unlikely unless it is good.

Otosclerosis causes a slowly progressive deafness, and the handicap is not usually noticeable until the hearing loss by air conduction has exceeded 30 decibels. By the time it reaches 60 decibels, the handicap is serious.

The ideal case for surgery, then, is one in which the hearing by bone conduction (and therefore the cochlear function) remains good (not more than 15–20 decibels of hearing loss), and the loss of hearing by air conduction is between 30 and 60 decibels. Theoretically, the hearing can never be raised above the level of the bone conduction loss so that the gain can never be greater than the difference—or 'gap'—between the hearing by bone conduction and that by air conduction. But if the obstruction can be successfully overcome, or the oval window re-opened, this 'bone-air gap' can be closed (Figure 15.3).

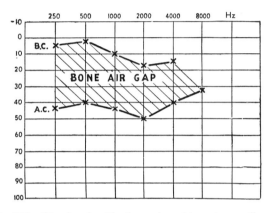

Fig. 15.3   Otosclerosis—The 'bone-air gap' (pure tone audiogram).

The history of this form of surgery starts with Kessel who, in 1876, first attempted to re-mobilize the fixed stapes in cases of otosclerosis. This manoeuvre was practised by many otologists during the ten-year period between 1880 and 1890, but the all-too-frequent occurrence of severe infection led to its abandonment. Surgeons then began to wonder whether there was any chance of creating a new window (or fenestra) into the inner ear, to take the place of the diseased, oval window in which the stapes was becoming increasingly fixed; and the first attempt to create such a new fenestra was made by Passow, in 1897. But it was not until 1913 that Bárány established a definitive operative technique. Jenkins, in the following year, was the first British otologist to perform the fenestration operation; he used a dental burr to drill an opening into the horizontal semicircular canal (page 110 and Figure 15.4) and he covered the new window with a skin graft. But perhaps the greatest names in the history of the fenestration operation are those of Holmgren, in Stockholm; Sourdille, in Paris; and Lempert, in New York.

Holmgren deserves special mention because it was he who amongst other things, first used a binocular dissecting microscope, in 1917; and there can be no doubt that the microscope is equalled in importance only by antibiotics and anaesthetics in the development of modern ear surgery. Sourdille was the first to obtain lasting results from fenestration surgery, in 1928; but it was Lempert who really popularized the operation, ten years later, when he described a practical, one-stage operation and published some very satisfactory results.

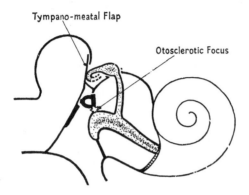

Fig. 15.4   The fenestration operation. The bony casing of the horizontal semicircular canal has been removed. So also have the incus, and the head and neck of the malleus. The handle of the malleus remains attached to the tympanic membrane which, together with the skin of the deeper parts of the external auditory canal, forms a 'tympano-meatal flap'. This flap is laid over the membranous semicircular duct and makes contact with it. This creates a 'new oval window' (the fenestra nov-ovalis), and there are now two functioning windows—the 'new oval window' and the round window.

The fenestration operation became rapidly popular in Britain soon after the Second World War, thanks very largely to the work of Cawthorne and Garnett-Passe in London, both now deceased and Simson Hall in Edinburgh.

The fenestration operation. In cases of otosclerosis, the 'differential' between the two windows which separate the air in the middle ear cavity from the fluids in the inner ear is reduced simply because the upper one, the oval window, is gradually closed off by the bony disease-process. The fenestration operation aimed at creating a new window, and the horizontal semicircular canal was chosen by the surgeon because it offered him the most ready access to the soft, membranous inner tube of the inner ear (the horizontal semicircular duct). Although many of us have come to think of the inner ear as consisting of two rather distinct parts—a hearing part, the cochlea; and a balancing part, the semicircular canals—we must remember (page 13) that all parts of the membranous tubular system of the inner ear are in direct continuity, structurally and (to some extent) functionally. Hence sound waves reaching the new fenestra could be transmitted through the fluids of the inner ear to the still-functioning round window (Figure 15.4).

Not every fenestration operation was initially successful and it had to be explained to the patient that, even with the most careful selection of cases and a perfect technique, not more than three in every four patients who were regarded as suitable were likely to experience a really appreciable immediate gain in hearing, to the level where they could enjoy the usual round of daily activities without the help of a hearing aid. After a year or two, this was reduced to a half of all the suitable cases; and as time went by more and more cases failed gradually, so that ultimately in most cases the hearing, though initially improved in many, returned to the pre-operative level. Vertigo (giddiness) was always troublesome for the first few days, although it usually responded readily to sedation and special exercises. Sometimes, however, it persisted for many months, especially in nervous patients.

Furthermore, the operation cavity often discharged persistently for weeks, or months, or even for years.

As it became increasingly obvious that the long-term results of the fenestration operation were extremely disappointing, nothing could have been more welcome than a less serious operation that was free from these defects; and a new phase in the surgery of otosclerosis was opened up by the work of Rosen, who shifted the attack back to the stapes itself.

The operation for mobilizing the stapes. It was in 1952 that Rosen first described a method of palpating the stapes to determine the degree of its fixation. Although this was designed primarily as a test of suitability (or otherwise) for the fenestration operation, he added that 'manipulation of the partially fixed stapes could result in further mobility of the footplate, with improved hearing'. This was, in fact, the first hint of a reversion to the stapes mobilization of Kessel, first suggested three-quarters of a century earlier.

In the following year Rosen described a technique of stapes mobilization, by moving the neck of the stapes in the direction of the stapedius tendon (Figure 2.3). This he called the 'indirect' method (Figure 15.5). At the time he published this paper, he had followed up 5 cases for periods ranging from 9 weeks to 1 year, and the hearing had returned almost to normal in two of them, improving in all. There was no post-operative vertigo; the patients spent only one day in hospital, and a fenestration operation was still possible if mobilization failed. He had followed up these five original cases, and added a further 20, when he published a further report with Bergman a year later. The hearing had been maintained in his earlier cases, and he had obtained a high proportion of satisfactory results in the later ones.

There were, however, some cases in which the stapes was too rigidly fixed in the oval window to be mobilized at the level of its neck, without

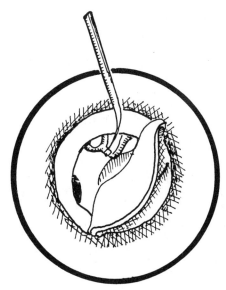

Fig. 15.5   Mobilization of the stapes—the indirect method. The stapes is mobilized at its neck.

a serious risk of fracturing the crura. Rosen therefore devised a new 'direct' method (Figure 15.6) in which the mobilizing force was applied directly to the footplate itself.

Rosen himself claimed that the results of stapes mobilization were as good as those of fenestration and in 1957 two French surgeons, Portmann and Claverie, reported an appreciable gain in hearing in no less than 48 of the 60 patients in whom they had performed the operation.

But sometimes the footplate of the stapes was so firmly fixed that all attempts to free it were doomed to failure. And the very nature of the underlying pathological process is such that further progression of the bony disease was to be expected in many cases. Indeed it happened; and the long-term results of stapes mobilization were never as good as those of the fenestration operation.

New and exciting possibilities were opened up, however, when it was suggested that hearing might be restored in cases of otosclerosis by *removal* of the stapes.

Removal of the stapes (stapedectomy). In 1958, J.J. Shea junior, of Memphis, described several cases of otosclerosis in which he had removed the stapes in its entirety. This, of course, left the oval window wide open, and the chain of ossicles disrupted. He closed the window with a vein graft, and bridged the gap between the window and the lenticular process of the incus with a tiny strut of polythene, a relatively

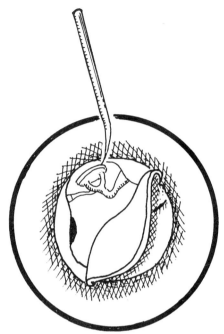

Fig. 15.6   Mobilization of the stapes—the direct method. The stapes is mobilized at its footplate.

inert material (Figure 15.7, A). In one of his earliest papers he reported (with Ewert) 94 successful results in a consecutive series of 100 of these operations.

Two years later Harold F. Schuknecht, now of Boston, devised a modification of Shea's original technique in which a fat-and-wire prosthesis (Figure 15.7, B) was placed between the incus and the oval window, the fat occupying the window, the wire being crimped (for extra security) over the lower end of the long process of the incus.

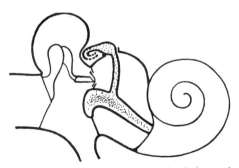

Fig. 15.7A.   Stapedectomy, with vein and polythene tube (Shea).

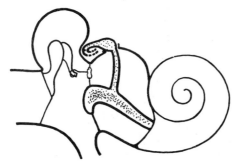

Fig 15.7 B.   Stapedectomy, with fat and wire (Schuknecht).

In terms of the hearing result, there was little if anything to choose between these two techniques, and the individual surgeon's choice was one of personal preference. But some authorities, notably Michel Portmann of Bordeaux, felt that, if possible, one should avoid the insertion of foreign materials into the ear; and he described, in 1961, a technique in which he kept intact the stapes superstructure (the head, neck and crura) and the joint between the incus and the stapes, thus preserving the blood supply to those structures. In this method the crura were detached from the footplate, and moved to one side while the whole or a part of the footplate was removed. A piece of vein was then used to cover the resultant aperture in the oval window, and the crura were finally replaced in their normal alignment, over the vein graft. Excellent results have been claimed, but most otologists have felt that its technical difficulty is not justified by any superiority of results.

Basically, however with relatively minor modifications, these three remained the standard methods of stapedectomy until 1963, when Shea devised a piston (Figure 15.7, c) made of the plastic material

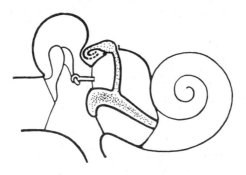

Fig. 15.7 C.   Stapedectomy, with Teflon piston (Shea).

Teflon. He had found that there was a small number of cases in which the footplate of the stapes was so grossly thickened by the invasion of otosclerotic bone that it was impossible to remove it, either in whole or in part, by the manipulation of simple dental-type instruments. In these cases, the oval window can be opened only by drilling; and the very limited field of operation will permit only of the use of an extremely fine drill, for all these procedures are carried out through an ordinary speculum, such as those which are used to examine the ear. The tiny hole that is made through the thick footplate in such cases is no bigger than 1 millimetre in diameter, and there is a greater risk of irreparable damage to the inner ear when a drill has to be used. Shea's Teflon piston had a diameter of only eight-tenths of a millimetre, and it can be fitted into this small hole, the outer 'hook' of the piston being subsequently fitted over the long process of the incus.

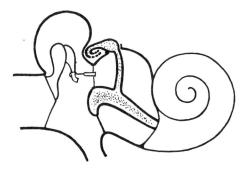

Fig. 15.7 D.   Stapedectomy, with stainless steel piston (McGee).

McGee designed a piston made of stainless steel (Figure 15.7, D), in which the hook is crimped in position over the incus with special forceps after carefully placing the far end of the piston into the oval window. There are other pistons which combine a 'body' of Teflon with a hook of stainless steel.

These piston techniques have proved extremely satisfactory, not only in these difficult cases of 'obliterative' otosclerosis in which only a part of the footplate is removed, but also in those cases where all of it is removed. Many otologists, including the present author, have adopted one or other of these piston methods as the standard form of stapedectomy, since it is the only technique which is applicable to every operable case of otosclerosis. But the method used still remains very much a matter of personal choice, and many otological surgeons now prefer, when possible, to remove the whole footplate, to cover the open oval window with a graft of some natural material and then to insert a prosthesis from the incus on to the graft.

Stapedectomy is not without its problems. And the greatest of these is the 'dead' ear. This is a calamity in which all hearing may be lost, sometimes months or years after the operation, and usually for no apparent reason. Cases have been reported in which a 'dead' ear has developed after stapedectomy in the *un*operated ear, and this of course suggests that this great misfortune is not necessarily related directly or indirectly, to the surgery.

However, the overall results of stapedectomy have been exceptionally gratifying, in the very great majority of cases, throughout the period of almost twenty years since its inception; and furthermore they have been maintained for much longer than those of the earlier operations of fenestration and stapes mobilization, which it has now entirely superseded.

It would now seem that stapedectomy has almost certainly come to stay—at least until such time as otosclerosis may be relieved by non-surgical means.

The surgery of otosclerosis represents one of the most important and dramatic advances in surgery over the last quarter of a century.

The surgery of chronic middle ear suppuration

Not so dramatic, nor yet so successful as the operations for otosclerosis, are the various operations on the sound-conducting apparatus which are now being used almost routinely in cases of chronic suppurative otitis media.

It remains as essential as ever, in the treatment of this condition, to eradicate all traces of disease from any part of the middle ear cleft that may be affected. But there are now available many methods of reconstructing an efficient sound conducting apparatus, after the excisive surgery has been completed, either at the same time or as a delayed second-stage operation.

The simplest of these methods is the repair of a tympanic membrane which has a central 'safe' perforation, the ossicular chain being intact. This operation was first performed by Berthold in 1878, and he gave to it the name of *Myringoplasty*.

Myringoplasty. It has already been said that a perforation may sometimes heal after the application of a caustic to its edges, but this is unlikely to be achieved with large perforations. Newer and much more certain methods are now used for the closure of these larger perforations (and some smaller ones) with grafts, after freshening the edges of the perforation and preparing a satisfactory bed for the graft to 'take' on. This operation has been widely criticized on the grounds that one can never be certain of the extent of the disease which may lie behind the perforation and, once it is closed, one has no further 'port-hole' for inspection. But Stuart Mawson came to its defence in the relatively early days of its revival. 'Myringoplasty,' he said, 'is a simple operation reserved for large dry residual perforations without active middle ear disease. ... It is a direct successor of older methods of patching holes in the membrane such as with cigarette paper, gold foil, or human amniotic membrane. ... Closure of a large perforation with free ... graft can be achieved in a high proportion of cases provided reinfection is eliminated, and only a third of my cases have failed to gain any improvenent in hearing.' Even if there is no improvement in the hearing (which is often very good, anyway, in these cases) Mawson believed that 'there is a definite place for attempting to close large dry perforations, by the simple expedient of skin grafting, without intending to do more than close the defect. ... ' (Figure 15.8). That was in

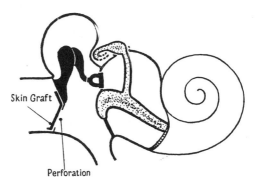

Fig. 15.8   Myringoplasty. The graft is placed over the denuded margin of the perforation, and the neighbouring depths of the external canal.

1957, when skin was used almost universally in these cases; but this became gradually replaced by *temporal fascia,* the covering of the temporal muscle just above the ear. This is still, at the time of writing, the most widely used material for grafting, but during the past 10 years there have been some encouraging results reported upon the use of whole drumheads removed from cadavers and stored for later use. These *tympanic homografts* were first described by J. Marquet, of Antwerp, in 1966; and theoretically they would seem to be the most natural form of replacement for a defective tympanic membrane, especially when the perforation is very large; but they have not found general favour, and fascial grafts are still used by most otological surgeons.

If we accept the well-established clinical concept of the safe ear, then we must believe that there is a place for myringoplasty. It may be requested by young men wishing to enter the armed services, or by those who cannot swim without re-infecting the ear.

Of course, hearing can only be significantly improved by simple myringoplasty if the ossicular chain is intact and functioning, and one must generally suspect a lesion of the chain if the hearing loss by air conduction exceeds 30–35 decibels.

Improvements in the technique of myringoplasty have brought with them a steady improvement in its functional results, especially in cases of traumatic perforation; but it must be remembered that it is applicable mainly to the inactive ear with a perforation that has remained dry for a long time, preferably for at least 6 months. Nor must we forget that this relatively simple procedure may be complicated, fortunately only rarely, by the so-called 'dead' ear, in which all hearing may be permanently lost.

Tympanoplasty. It is common knowledge to any otologist of experience that hearing will sometimes improve when suppuration is active; that is to say, the patient may hear better when the ear is discharging than when it is dry. It has also been known for many years that hearing could be improved artificially, and sometimes quite dramatically, by the simple expedient of loading or shielding the round window by the introduction of a pledglet of cotton-wool saturated with liquid paraffin and placed over the niche of the round window. Furthermore, hearing has sometimes improved after radical operations on the middle ear and mastoid, even after the most extensive surgery; but just as frequently, if not more so, the hearing has been worse after such operations, and it was not until the German otologists Wullstein and Zöllner related their experiences and observations that otologists become aware of the reasons for these well-known but hitherto unexplained phenomena.

Zöllner, in 1955, described the case of a man who suffered a traumatic rupture of the tympanic membrane. The incudo-stapedial joint was destroyed and the stapes could be seen through the perforation. The remains of the tympanic membrane adhered only to the lower part of the middle ear cavity, including the region of the round window, which thus became separated from the oval window and the isolated stapes (Figures 15.9 and 15.10). Now, the interesting part of the story is that this man's hearing was practically normal despite the extensive destruction of the middle ear structures; and Zöllner believed that this astonishingly good hearing must have resulted from the acoustic separation of the two windows. 'Such spontaneous plastic results,' he observed, 'are sometimes found after inflammatory lesions and radical operations. Observation of these facts and the good hearing resulting induced me to create similar conditions artificially by means of plastic measures.' and so was born the principle of the 'differential' and the operation of tympanoplasty.

There are several types of tympanoplasty, but whatever type is used, the first essential is to remove all diseased tissues completely and meticulously. When this has been done we can take stock of the state of the ossicular chain.

Wullstein (in 1953) formulated several principles of tympanoplasty, and he described five operative types; a sixth type (sono-inversion)

was added later (in 1961) by the Spanish otologist Garcia-Ibañez. These are shown in Figure 15.11.

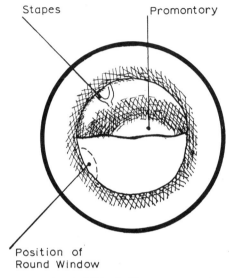

Fig. 15.9 'Nature's tympanoplasty' (Zöllner). The stapes remains mobile and is 'acoustically separated' from the round window (indicated by the dotted line), by the adhesion to the promontory of the remains of the tympanic membrane.

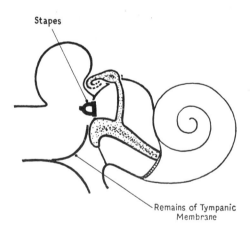

Fig. 15.10 The 'baffle effect' of 'Nature's tympanoplasty'.

Of Wullstein's five types, Type I was the simple myringoplasty, described in (Figure 15.11, A). Type II involved a repair of the drumhead, and covering of a relatively intact ossicular chain with

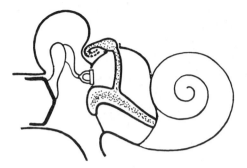

Fig. 15.11   Types of tympanoplasty.
A, Type I (Wullstein).

the graft (Figure 15.11, B). Type III tympanoplasty was applied to cases in which the malleus and incus had been removed by surgery or by disease, the stapes remaining intact and mobile (Figure 15.11, C). In birds, a single strut of bone—the columella—takes the place of the human chain of ossicles, and it transmits sounds direct from the

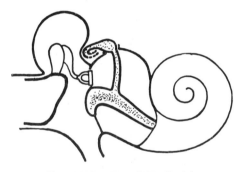

Fig. 15.11 B.   Type II (Wullstein).

tympanic membrane to the labyrinthine window. In this type of operation—the so-called 'columella' type—the graft is made to lie over, and make contact with the stapes, thus simulating the columella of birds.

The Type IV operation was applicable when the ossicular chain was disrupted and the stapes was also deficient. Under the circumstances it was impossible to achieve the columella effect. The object of this type of operation was to restore the differential between the two windows by leaving the oval window exposed in the operation cavity, and by placing a baffle over the round window, to prevent sound waves from reaching it direct, and to separate it acoustically from the oval window (Figure 15.11, D). A graft was applied to the bared promontory and to the lower half of the circumference of the deep external auditory canal. This left an air space between the upper

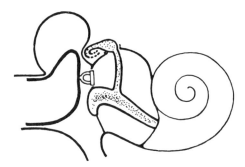

Fig. 15.11 C.   Type III (Wullstein).

orifice of the Eustachian tube and the round window, so recreating a minor middle ear cavity which communicated with the nasopharynx through a normally-functioning Eustachian tube. It will be noticed that this state of affairs approximated very closely to that described by Zöllner in the case of the man who had had a traumatic rupture.

In Type V tympanoplasty, the graft was placed over a fenestration of the horizontal semicircular canal, in cases in which the footplate was fixed (Figure 15.11, E). Finally Garcia-Ibañez added a Type VI

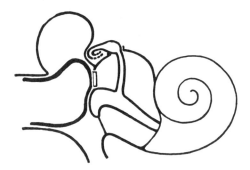

Fig. 15.11 D.   Type IV (Wullstein).

operation (Figure 15.11, F) in which sound protection was provided for the oval window, and the niche of the round window was left uncovered so that it might receive the direct impact of the sound waves.

These principles looked simple enough, and for several years these operations were increasingly performed by otologists throughout the world. But early optimism was not justified by the longer-term results and many surgeons, disappointed and disillusioned, began to abandon them. Fortunately, however, studies continued and, little by little, new principles began to emerge.

In the first place, it was recognized that a thin mobile drumhead was essential, an intact one preferable, for a successful outcome.

Secondly, it became clear that, in order to transmit sounds from this new membrane to the inner ear, an intact mobile ossicular chain was also required.

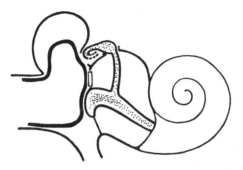

Fig. 15.11 E.   Type V (Wullstein).

Thirdly, it became increasingly evident, as time went by, that many of the long-term failures of early tympanoplastic surgery were caused by failure of the reconstituted drumhead to maintain sufficient tension —with its subsequent collapse and the virtual obliteration of an air-filled middle ear cavity.

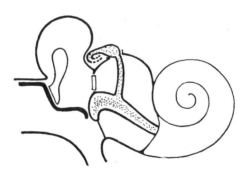

Fig. 15.11 F.   Sound inversion (Garcia-Ibañez).

And finally—and this goes almost without saying—there must be a functioning Eustachian tube to replace the air in the cavity; and a healthy lining throughout the middle ear cleft.

To take the last of these requirements first, it is fortunately true to say that in most of these cases, tubal function is in fact normal; but unfortunately, there is not uncommonly some residual inflammation in the mucous membrane of the middle ear. And it is essential to remove any obstruction and to eliminate any infection from the upper respiratory tract (including its extensions into the middle ear cleft) before directing any surgical attack towards the ear itself.

In the early days of tympanoplasty, the problem of creating a thin mobile tympanic membrane was brought about, at least in part, by the almost universal practice of using skin as the grafting material. For skin lies unhappily in the ear, and after many hundreds and even thousands of apparently successful initial results, these grafts began to break down and finally to perish. And just as this problem seemed to have been very largely overcome by the substitution of connective tissue (particularly the readily accessible temporal fascia) for skin, so Marquet (a Belgian otologist) came along with the idea of a *tympanic homograft* (see Myringoplasty, page 118).

A much more difficult problem is the restoration of a mobile functioning ossicular chain. Many artificial prostheses—of several materials (mainly metal or plastic) and of various shapes and sizes (such as simple struts, pistons, or even 'clothes pegs')—have been applied with ingenuity to the restoration of continuity, in those ossicular defects which are commonly associated with chronic middle ear disease. But however inert these materials may appear to be, the tendency now is to use natural rather than foreign materials; and there is a growing tendency to use the patient's own ossicles or their remains, especially the incus or malleus, or the ossicles removed from a cadaver and stored, to be used later as an *ossicular homograft*.

If, for example, the incus is dislocated or its long process is eroded by disease, it may be removed and 'transposed' between the stapes (if the latter is mobile) and the malleus (Figure 15.12, A). And if the crura of the stapes are also missing, the incus may be removed and replaced in the ear in such a way that its short process rests on the mobile footplate of the stapes, and its articular facet (which normally articulates with the head of the malleus) can be wedged behind the malleus (Figure 15.12, B). These are two types of *incus transposition*. Alternatively and increasingly, *malleus homografts* are being used.

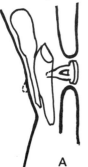
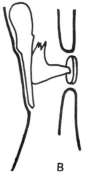

Fig. 15.12   Incus transposition.
A, Type 1.   B, Type 2.

By far the most difficult ossicular defect to overcome is one in which the handle of the malleus is missing, and this is usually associated with destruction of the incus, and sometimes also of the stapes super-structure. In such cases it may be possible to use a homograft of the tympanic membrane, with the malleus and incus attached to it—followed later, at a second-stage operation, by stapedectomy or preferably by the interposition of wire between the incus and the mobile footplate. This is known as a *middle ear transplant*.

Many of these operations are still in their surgical 'childhood', and time alone will permit us to evaluate their true eventual value. There is no doubt, however, that they represent a genuine and major advance.

The older formulae of Wullstein's original five types of tympano-plasty have now been replaced by the much simpler one: Tympanoplasty = Myringoplasty + Ossiculoplasty; but problems still remain, and one of the most difficult of these is to be found in patients who have had previous radical mastoid operations or one of its several modifications. These old and well-established operations may still be necessary in many cases, but they involve the removal of a part, and sometimes of a very large part, of the posterior bony wall of the external auditory canal. And much attention is now being given to preservation of the entire bony wall of the canal, or to its reconstruction in those who have already had previous radical surgery.

'Combined approach' tympanoplasty is one such operation in which preservation of an intact canal wall is achieved by combining one approach to the middle ear through the canal itself (anterior tympano-tomy) with another through the mastoid from behind (posterior tympanotomy). Alternatively, in patients in whom the posterior canal wall has been removed by previous surgery, attempts are now frequently made to reconstitute the wall by replacing 'wedges' of bone from the mastoid cortex or by a variety of other techniques. In theory at least, these operations allow of better placement of the grafts, and better tension within them. However there are serious doubts in the minds of many otologists about the possibility of eradicating all disease effectively and permanently without removing at least a part of the bony canal wall, and disturbing reports are appearing about an unexpectedly high rate of recurrence of disease, and especially of cholesteatoma, some years after apparently successful surgery.

New techniques are constantly evolving, and it is to be hoped that the future will witness the solution to some of the many problems which still exist.

The surgery of traumatic ossicular lesions

Most of the rather rare traumatic lesions of the auditory ossicles can be corrected surgically by a variety of ossiculoplastic procedures, some of them very ingenious. These operations make use of the principles and practice of stapedial and tympanoplastic surgery.

Details of technique would be out of place in a monograph of this sort; but it may be said in general that, whereas some cases can be satisfactorily treated by the use of artificial prostheses, other cases are more suitable for the use of natural materials such as bone and connective tissue, or incus or malleus homografts.

As in tympanoplasty, there is a growing tendency amongst otologists to show a preference for natural over foreign materials.

16. The Deaf Child

The causes of congenital deafness

There is a very small number of children who are born deaf because the conducting apparatus has failed to develop in part or in whole. At one end of the scale, there may be only a simple plug of solid tissues occluding the outer part of the external auditory canal; at the other extreme, it may remain uncanalized throughout the whole of its length and the ossicles may be ill-developed or malformed.

These congenital lesions of the conducting mechanism may be associated with other defects, as in the *Treacher-Collins syndrome,* (Figure 16.1) in which the deafness is associated with a typical 'fish-face' deformity, due to under-development of the lower jaws and certain of the facial bones (mandibular facial dysostosis). Congenital

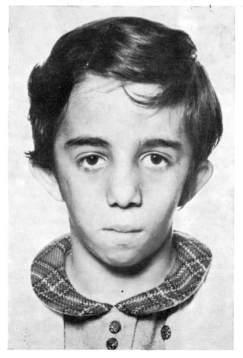

Fig. 16.1   Treacher-Collins syndróme (see text).

conductive deafness also occurs in some children who have been born with limb deformities due to the ingestion by the mother during pregnancy of the notorious drug *thalidomide*. Some of these defects may be correctable by surgery.

For practical purposes, however, the vast majority of all children born deaf are born with some defect of the sensori-neural apparatus and such defects may be caused either by failure of development before birth or by damage to the cochlea or the auditory nerve at or about the time of birth.

It is customary to consider the causes of congenital sensori-neural deafness in a chronological sequence and they fall into three main groups: the *hereditary* group, due to genetic influences; the *pre-natal* group, due to a variety of noxious influences upon the developing embryo; and the *perinatal* group, due to any one of a number of 'accidents' at the time of birth itself, shortly before birth, or within the earliest hours or days after birth.

Dr Lindsey Batten, speaking to the Section of General Practice at the Royal Society of Medicine in March 1957, described these three groups as the 'Bad Seed', the 'Damaged Embryo', and the 'Pressure Group'. This latter term would seem to be too restrictive for the important perinatal group, and the term 'Hazardous Birth' might give a more all-embracing conception of the dangers of being born.

The hereditary group – the 'bad seed'. The incidence of hereditary congenital deafness is determined by Mendelian law, and transmission of this type of deafness may be either *dominant* or *recessive*. In dominant transmission in which only one of the parents need carry the affected gene, the chances of the offspring being affected is as high as 50 per cent. On the other hand, in the recessive type in which both parents must be carriers of the particular gene, only 25 per cent of the offspring are affected. The former mode of transmission accounts for approximately 10 per cent of cases of hereditary congenital deafness, the latter for the remaining majority of about 90 per cent. And the hereditary group as a whole probably accounts for one-third of all cases of congenital deafness.

It has, of course, been known for a very long time that many cases of congenital deafness have a strong tendency to occur in families and that congenital deafness may be associated with other congenital defects; but recent research has brought to light several conditions in which deafness forms but a part of a syndrome, or symptom-complex, hitherto unrecognized. And if we add these syndromes—as we must—to the present group of hereditary cases, it will be evident that the 'bad seed' must be responsible for many more cases of congenital deafness. Such a combination of symptoms was described by Waardenburg in 1951 and their association with deafness was emphasized by the work of Dr L. Fisch, Otologist to the Nuffield

Hearing and Speech Centre attached to the Institute of Laryngology and Otology in London.

A prominent fold of skin at the inner angles of the eyes (the epicanthal fold) gives the impression of a broad nasal bridge and widely-spaced eyes; the eyes may be of different colours (heterochromia iridium)—one blue and one brown, for example; and there is often a broad streak of white hair right in the middle of the forehead. One or more of these symptoms—without deafness—may occur in one or more members of each generation, sometimes for many generations, until—for no apparent reason—a child is born deaf. This child may have none of the other clinical features of the syndrome and it may be only their occurrence in other members of his family that allows us to fit the deafness into the Waardenburg symptom-complex and hence to establish the case as one of hereditary type.

The pigmentary changes in the eyes and hair are of particular interest and Dr Fisch, in his further studies of this syndrome, found that the neural apparatus of the cochlea and all the pigments throughout the body share a common origin in the developing embryo—from the primitive 'neural crest'. He observed, furthermore, that they also share a common protective function throughout the animal kingdom.

Several other syndromes have come to light in which hereditary deafness occurs with a variety of pigmentary changes. One of the commonest of these is Usher's syndrome, in which the deafness is associated with the condition of retinitis pigmentosa and which accounts for about one-tenth of all cases of recessive hereditary deafness. Retinitis pigmentosa is a progressive degenerative lesion of the inner layer of the retina of the eye, in which the visual fields gradually contract and night blindness ultimately follows. Pigment is deposited in spidery forms in the periphery of the eye. The hearing loss affects the high tones first, but it develops late in the disease, after the visual fields have narrowed. Deafness occurs in between a fifth and a quarter of all cases of retinitis pigmentosa, but it is seen much more commonly in some families than in others. The combination of retinitis pigmentosa with hereditary nerve deafness, usually recessive, may also occur in a variety of other syndromes—notably in association with obesity, dwarfism and mental retardation.

W. Tietz, in 1960, described a syndrome in which inherited deafness was associated with albinism, in which there is a generalized loss of pigment, rather than a localized loss as in Waardenburg's syndrome. The eyebrows are absent, the irises blue. There is said to be a high incidence of this syndrome in Israel, especially in males.

Working in the same Unit and at the same time as Fisch was working on the Waardenburg syndrome—but quite independently—the present writer was investigating a group of cases of congenital deafness in which the hearing loss was progressive and affected mainly the high tones at first. It so happened—by pure coincidence—that three of these children presented themselves at one and the same clinic, on one and the same afternoon; and two other features were seen in all of them—they all had blonde hair and they all had blue eyes. These pigmentary changes have since been seen on many occasions in children with progressive high-tone deafness and in some of them a similar deafness had been known to exist in other members of the family.

The interest of seeing a brother and sister together not long after this association had been noticed—both with blonde hair and both with blue eyes—was surpassed only by the excitement of seeing a father and daughter with the same gold and silver hair and the same steely blue eyes. The father was already known to have had a progressive high-tone deafness of many years' standing (Figure 16.2, A), and the daughter's hearing loss was just becoming apparent (Figure

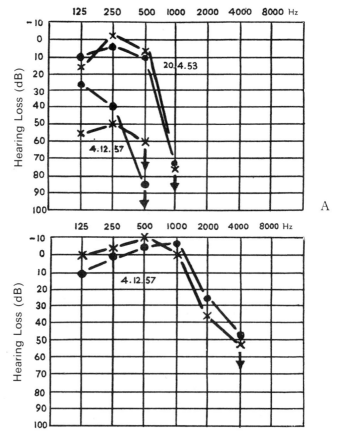

Fig. 16.2   Familial progressive high-tone deafness. (Pure tone audiograms) A, Father. B, Daughter (see text).

16.2, B), Many months later the father wrote to me: 'I have also traced that an elderly aunt (on my father's side) became progressively deaf, and strange to say I can see certain similarities between this lady, Angela (the daughter) and myself.' My interest in this symptom-complex (in over a dozen cases) was heightened by an article in one of our more prominent Sunday newspapers on 'an unsuspected 'metabolic' disorder called phenylketonuria'. These children,' said the Medical Correspondent, 'frequently have ash-grey hair.'

Turning to the most recent textbook on Paediatrics, I learnt that this 'phenylketonuria' was an inborn error of metabolism associated with mental deficiency; that the hair is often 'strikingly fair' and the eyes are usually blue; that certain biochemical changes occur, the effect of which is a failure to form the chemical substance 'tyrosine' from another chemical (phenylalanine); and that this 'tyrosine' (which is not formed as it should be) is a precursor of 'melanin'—a pigment. It is interesting that there is also a defect in the metabolism of tyrosine in Tietz's syndrome.

No sooner had my interest in these biochemical changes been aroused than an article appeared in the *Lancet* (in March 1958) in which Doctors Morgans and Trotter described the cases of 'two siblings . . . in whom nerve deafness present from birth was associated with a goitre developing during childhood'. These authors described the syndrome as one of 'genetic and biochemical interest'. It is generally known as Pendred's syndrome, and it is thought that the deafness and the goitre are independent manifestations of the same recessive genetic defect. It has been estimated that 10 per cent of all cases of recessive hereditary sensori-neural deafness are due to this relatively common disorder, in which there is an abnormal metabolism of iodine. The thyroid enlargement appears during childhood and it may vary in size, becoming nodular in adult life; the deafness is usually congenital, but cases have been recorded in which the deafness has started after the age of four years. The administration of desiccated thyroid extract is effective in decreasing the goitre, but unfortunately it does not affect the hearing.

There are several other syndromes in which inherited deafness is associated with various disturbances of metabolism—Hurler's syndrome, with a disturbance of 'muco-poly-saccharide' metabolism; Tay-Sachs disease, with a disturbance of lipid metabolism; and Wilson's disease, with a disturbance of copper metabolism.

In Hurler's syndrome, a recessive sensori-neural deafness is associated with 'gargoylism', a condition in which the head is large, the face is flat and ugly, the neck is short, the eyes are enlarged and wide apart, the teeth are widely spaced and the abdomen is protruding. The deafness is usually profound and progressive, usually after speech has begun. It is preceded by mental deficiency, dwarfism and enlargement of the spleen and liver. The disease is usually fatal.

In Tay-Sachs disease, a high frequency deafness is associated with 'amaurotic family idiocy', in which there is an arrest in general development, with progressive loss of vision, seizures, wasting, dementia and finally a fatal outcome.

In Wilson's disease, the deafness is accompanied by ascites (fluid in the abdomen), jaundice, enlargement of spleen and liver, fixed unblinking stare, gaping mouth, tremor, seizures and dementia. The onset of symptoms may occur at any time between 5 and 40 years of age.

In addition to these various metabolic disorders, there are two further syndromes worthy of note: Alport's syndrome and the Klippel-Feil syndrome. The former is characterized by sensori-neural deafness, usually progressive, associated with symptomless haematuria and albuminuria (blood and albumin in the urine); these may occur in the first week of life, but it is not until the second decade that high blood pressure and renal failure occur; male patients, who are worse affected, usually die of chronic nephritis before the age of 30. In the latter syndrome, nerve deafness is associated with a very short, stiff neck and a hairline extending down to the back.

It is becoming more and more apparent that hereditary nerve deafness may result from many different genetic abnormalities, which may cause widely divergent errors of metabolism, with resultant damage to the organ of hearing. According to the particular metabolic disturbance operating in any particular syndrome, the effect on hearing may be immediate or delayed, thus explaining why hereditary nerve deafness is not always congenital.

All very fascinating so far, but where do we go from here? What, for instance, is the connection (if any) between the pigmentary changes of the Waardenburg syndrome and the blue-eyed blondes who suffer from progressive high-tone deafness? And where the connection between these latter children and those other blue-eyed blondes (the 'phenylketonurics') whose mental deficiency is now thought to be due to biochemical changes? And can these changes be correlated in any way with those other biochemical changes which occur in the children with congenital deafness and goitre?

All these questions await solution and much more research is required, but it is to be hoped that the day will not be too distant when the closer liaison of the otologist with the geneticist and the biochemist may bring forth the answer. At least one can say, with some confidence, that more and more is being learnt, slowly but surely, about several new syndromes—each of them taking us a little nearer to a fuller understanding of the problem of hereditary congenital deafness—a condition in which we have all felt so helpless so far.

The pre-natal group—the 'damaged embryo'. In 1945 Carruthers reported the occurrence of congenital deafness as a sequel to maternal rubella, and doctors have since shown serious concern about the possible dangers (to the developing embryo) of other noxious influences.

Rubella (German measles) will cause congenital deafness, not infrequently progressive, only if it is contracted by the mother during the first three or four months of her pregnancy. Thereafter, the neural structures of the embryonic cochlea are more or less fully developed and appear to be almost immune from the toxic effects of the rubella virus. In normal times as many as 10 per cent of all cases of congenital deafness can be attributed to it; but Fisch has emphasized that after epidemics the proportion may be much higher. Other defects may also occur. It has been said that if rubella develops in the first month of pregnancy, one child in every two is likely to be handicapped—by deafness, blindness, heart disease or mental deficiency. This high incidence is reduced to one-in-four during the second month, one-in-six during the third.

Other viral infections, notably influenza, are thought to account for a small number of cases and it is also possible that certain drugs may damage the immature cochlea during the first three critical months of embryonic life. It is in this period, for example, that abortifacient drugs are sometimes used, and an unsuccessful attempt to terminate a pregnancy may lead to tragic consequences in the unwanted child.

Congenital syphilis is correctly included in this group because, although the symptom of deafness is rarely present at birth, the noxious influences of the syphilitic disease are transmitted from the infected mother to her child during her pregnancy. There is an early form, in which the deafness begins in the first two years of life; and a late form in which the deafness usually begins between the ages of eight and twenty, not uncommonly at about the time of puberty.

The perinatal group—the 'hazardous birth'. The perinatal period is a somewhat ill-defined period of a few days—possibly a week or so—around and about the time of birth. It includes the period immediately before birth, the moment of birth itself and a short period immediately after birth. Toxaemias in the later stages of pregnancy; prematurity; birth injury, instrumental or accidental; anoxia, or lack of oxygen; and neo-natal jaundice are all numbered amongst the perinatal causes of congenital deafness.

Perhaps the most interesting of these conditions is the neo-natal jaundice caused by an incompatibility (between mother and child) of the Rhesus blood groups—so called because the initial work on these blood groups was carried out on the Rhesus monkey. In 1940 Landsteiner and Wiener demonstrated the presence of the Rhesus (or Rh) factor on the red blood cells of about 85 per cent of Europeans. The remaining 15 per cent whose red cells did not possess this factor were termed Rh negative.

If a Rhesus negative mother is carrying a Rhesus positive baby, the Rh factor (antigen) may pass from the child's blood, through the placenta, into the mother's circulation. Here antibodies are formed and they pass freely between the mother and her unborn child. Their concentration remains low in a first confinement but gradually increases with each succeeding pregnancy; and when it has risen beyond a certain critical point a reaction takes place between antigen and antibody. This causes a destruction of the child's red blood cells ('haemolysis') and releases a bile-pigment (bilirubin) into the child's bloodstream.

As long as he remains unborn, his mother's liver can dispose of the bilirubin; but as soon as he is parted from his mother's circulation, his own immature liver is unable to cope with it and its concentration rises in his own circulation. An excessive bilirubin concentration in the child's blood will cause a yellow staining of the skin (jaundice), and if his blood is not entirely replaced within a few hours of birth, the pigment may also penetrate the blood-brain barrier to cause a staining of certain nerve cells. These may include the cochlear nuclei (page   ). It is this kernicterus—literally a nuclear jaundice—which causes the deafness and other neurological complications of Haemolytic Disease of the Newborn. A similar kernicterus may also result from prematurity.

The deafness in these condtions is therefore not strictly congenital, but as these children have virtually no experience (and almost certainly no memory) of normal hearing, it is convenient clinically to think of their deafness as congenital rather than acquired.

Rhesus incompatibility is probably responsible for 2–3 per cent of all cases of deafness in infancy, and this proportion should be diminishing. But the perinatal group as a whole must account for about 20–25 per cent.

Unfortunately, it is still impossible to determine the cause of deafness in far too many children who are born deaf—at least 20 per cent at the most optimistic estimate and probably twice this number in most of the larger series of published cases. But this seemingly large gap is being gradually narrowed and it would be unwise to forget that very little was known about the causes of congenital deafness immediately before the Second World War beyond the fact that a few were due to congenital syphilis, and a rather larger number occurred in families. It was not until 1940 that the Rhesus blood groups were first described and a further ten years elapsed before their association with deafness was recognized. The war had almost finished when Carruthers, in Australia, described the deafness resulting from maternal rubella and recent work on hereditary deafness must surely help to close the gap still further.

Interesting and exciting possibilities are constantly presenting themselves to those engaged in research, and it is the earnest hope of all who work for the deaf child that more and more cases of congenital deafness will soon be preventable.

The site and extent of the damage – pathology

Pathology is the study of disease, and it behoves us at this point to say a few words about the various pathological changes which occur in congenital deafness. These changes may affect either the end-organ or the auditory nervous pathway.

It is the organ of Corti which is usually affected by genetic weakness, and the extent of the damage may vary from minor defects in the hair-cells to total absence of the cochlea.

In the pre-natal group, the development of the neural epithelium is arrested by the toxic effects of maternal rubella or other noxious influences, and the degree of this arrest is determined by the stage in embryonic life at which the mother is affected. It is greatest soon after conception but diminishes as the pregnancy advances. And since the cochlea is usually affected throughout its length, from base to apex, the hearing loss tends to be uniform for all frequencies.

In the perinatal group, however, the cochlea is normal and the site of the lesion is in the dorsal cochlear nuclei, particularly in those nerve cells which are concerned with the transmission of the higher frequencies. For this reason, the deafness which sometimes results from kernicterus, anoxia or birth injury tends to affect predominantly the high tones.

Deafness, of course, is never lethal and it will take many years to complete the pathological picture of congenital deafness. But great strides have been made in recent years and there can be little doubt that further knowledge in this field will lead to a greater understanding of the complex problems which confront the clinical otologist.

The diagnosis of congenital deafness

The history. The accurate assessment of hearing in young children is the highly specialized work of a team of experts, but much valuable information can be obtained from a careful and detailed history.

Congenital deafness most commonly presents itself through lack of response to speech or through lateness or defect in the child's own speech; and the hearing should be investigated with the utmost thoroughness in any child whose speech develops late or badly.

It is far too easy to assume that the late talker is 'just a bit slow', or to say that 'he'll be all right, his father didn't speak till he was four'. It is perfectly true, of course, that the backward child is late in talking and that there do appear to be some families in whom, for no apparent reason, speech develops late in several of its members and sometimes in several generations. It is also true that little or nothing can be done to hasten the speech of the backward child or the 'familial late-talker'. But herein lies the difference. Something can and should be done for the child whose speech is retarded by deafness, and his language can only be developed to its fullest potential if his handicap is recognized early and training begun without delay.

The defective speech of the partially hearing child is essentially a vowel speech, defective in the fainter, high-pitched consonant sounds. The extent of the defect will depend very largely on the nature and severity of the deafness (which also determine the age at which it is likely to be noticed) and may vary from a very marked defect, almost entirely devoid of consonants and usually noticed during the second year of life, to a minimal disturbance which may go quite unnoticed or be passed as normal childish speech until the child enters school. Particularly does this apply to cases of abrupt high-tone deafness, in which the cause of the speech disorder may not be recognized until the child is 7 or 8 years old, and in exceptional cases several years older.

It goes without saying that the more severe the deafness, the earlier is it likely to be detected by the parents. And in cases of total or sub-total deafness it is not uncommonly suspected within the first year—usually because the child shows none of the normal reactions to the many loud noises of everyday life; sometimes because 'he has always been so placid' or 'he seemed too good'. As in all other things, experience counts for much, and any mother will tend to recognize a relatively slight degree of deafness in her third or fourth child earlier than she would suspect a severer one in her first-born.

Many children who are born partially deaf learn to lip-read quite spontaneously. They 'listen with their eyes', and deafness should always be suspected in the child who looks with rapt attention at the speaker's lips.

When a mother thinks her child is deaf, she is very rarely wrong and it is unforgivable to dismiss a mother's convictions without a most careful and thorough examination of the hearing.

With the rare exception of congenital atresia of the external auditory canal, physical examination of the ears is entirely negative and X-rays are of limited value. Since the deafness is of the sensori-neural type in the vast majority of children born deaf their handicap can be diagnosed only by the functional examination of their hearing.

Diagnostic tests of hearing in infants and young children. In testing the hearing of adults, we ask them to tell us whether or not they hear certain sounds. It is obviously impossible to do this with infants and young children, and we must employ a variety of 'play' techniques in which the child is taught to *do* something, not to *say* something, every time he hears a sound. Before we can begin to undertake any such tests, we must have a clear understanding of the development of hearing and speech in the normally hearing child.

Attempts have been made, within the last fifteen years or so, to screen fetuses for their responses to sound, these responses being assessed as changes in heart rate or as movements occurring immediately after the onset of the stimulus, usually from a vibrator situated on the maternal abdomen immediately above the fetal head. Early work on the human fetus, notably by Doctors Murphy and Bench and their associates in Reading, was conducted *before term* by recordings made by way of the maternal body wall, the changes in heart rate being measured by recordings of the fetal electrocardiogram, the fetal movements being measured by recording the transient pressure changes in intra-uterine pressure caused by fetal activity. Advances in obstetrics now permit more direct recording *during birth* of the fetal heart rate and electroencephalograph (of 'brain waves') from electrodes on the fetal scalp.

The first requirement of all hearing tests in young children is a natural and friendly atmosphere, as far removed as possible from the hum-drum and hurly-burly of a busy hospital clinic. A separate room is essential and it should be effectively sound-proofed. Small tables and chairs must also be available, together with a good selection of toys and testing apparatus.

No child will co-operate fully until he has been allowed to settle in and one must be prepared to allow at least a half, often three-quarters, of an hour for each child at each attendance. Several attendances may be necessary, preferably at short intervals, before he has learnt to know his new friends and to enjoy the games he is asked to play with them. The interview can only be regarded as entirely satisfactory when the child is reluctant to leave at the end of it!

Some of the children who attend audiology clinics have already had experience of hospitals, and every doctor or nurse is likely to be associated with pain or discomfort. It is not surprising that the child's confidence in the 'man in white' is almost certainly undermined, and the team of an audiology unit should dress normally. 'No white coats' should be the rule.

It is of the utmost importance to establish *rapport* with every child and the first lesson to be learnt by those who are not familiar with the handling of children is that one must be prepared, quite literally, to get down to the child's own level—if necessary, on bended knees.

In performing full diagnostic tests of hearing, it is customary nowadays to start always with faint sounds; but the final range of testing sounds must depend ultimately on the degree of deafness and this can often be anticipated by careful attention to the details of the history. There can be no hard and fast rules about these things, but it is usually possible to make an intelligent guess at the likely extent of the handicap, and the choice of tests is based much more on experience than on any written formula. In describing these tests and the age at which they are used, it must be remembered that one is referring, not to the child's chronological age but to his mental age, and that the backward child will respond at a considerably lower level than the bright one. Within these defined limits, most of the tests of hearing in infants and young children can be said to fall broadly into one or other of two main groups—simple distraction techniques, and conditioning techniques.

Distraction techniques

It is rarely possible to train a child to perform a purposeful conditioned response to sound before the age of about 3 to $3\frac{1}{2}$. In children under this age we must therefore look for simpler responses.

In testing the small child, it is of the utmost importance that he should not be able to see or feel the source of the testing sound. The child who is deprived of hearing at, or soon after, birth will often develop his other senses to a remarkable degree and we must be careful not to cast shadows over him as we approach, nor to walk too heavily towards him lest he feel the vibrations from our feet. He may even turn to the odour of a highly scented hair-cream or face powder!

If the child is too young to walk, he should be seated on his mother's lap and allowed to settle down. Before the testing is begun, he must be distracted by his rattle or some other toy. If he is not distracted at all, he will tend to look round and watch the person who is going to test him; if he is distracted too much, he may become so engrossed in the game he is playing that he will not respond to sounds which are well within his hearing capacity. It is never easy to distract an infant just enough—not too little, not too much—but it is pointless to begin any formal testing until this point has been reached.

The new-born baby usually responds to loud sounds with the so-called Moro or 'startle' reflex, aptly described by Mary Sheridan as 'a sort of jerky extension of the spine and limbs, followed by a quick bowing movement of the arms over the chest, usually accompanied by a cry'. This general withdrawal response is in the nature of a primitive protective reflex and is common up to the age of about six months, but thereafter the child begins to localize sounds and commonly responds by a simple turning of the head towards their source. Once a response has been obtained, he should be shown the source of the noise, which should be pleasant to look at if possible; for at this age he is unlikely to repeat his responses unless he is interested in the sound source. Children with defective vision should be allowed to feel the testing objects, and they may tend to incline rather than turn their heads. Sometimes, however, the response is so slight that it can only be recognized by the highly skilled observer. The child may blink or his eyelids may open; occasionally he will give a faint smile, sometimes a frown; and not uncommonly, in the first year of life, the response is a 'negative' one, in so far as he will merely cease to do whatever he is doing—kicking, smiling, chuckling— at the moment when he hears the testing sound, or a few seconds later. Furthermore, at about the age of 1 many children will respond only once to any particular sound and the examiner must be prepared to change rapidly from one sound to another as the child loses interest in each of them, one by one. Perhaps the easiest time to test the infant is that short period of half-awareness when he is just about to wake from natural sleep.

Complex sound stimuli are more effective than pure tones in eliciting responses in infants between 0 and 6 months of age. Although such complex sounds as the crinkling of paper or the rattling of a spoon in a cup were previously employed as 'meaningful' sounds, Dr John Bench and his colleagues in Reading have shown that it is the 'frequency bandwidth' of such complex sounds which is of foremost importance in eliciting behavioural responses in infants of 1 week, 6 weeks and 6 months of age. Loud (90dB SPL) complex sounds are generally required for newborn and 6-week-old infants because they spend so much of their time asleep, but quieter (60dB) complex stimuli are more suitable for 6-month-old babies because they are conveniently tested when awake. The human voice is effective for testing 6-month-old babies, but not for 1 and 6-week-old infants. From the age of 5 or 6 months onwards, the alert baby is able, not only to detect a sound stimulus, but also to *localise* it, by turning his eye or his head towards its source.

There can be little doubt that the most difficult age is the age at which the child has just begun to walk and is beginning to explore his widening horizon. At this stage in his development, the examiner must be prepared to follow closely on his heels through all his wanderings, banging a drum or calling his name at any suitable moment that offers itself.

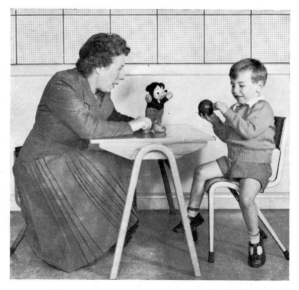

Fig. 16.3 A

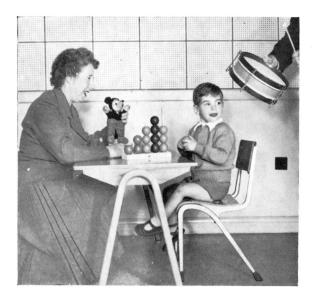

Fig. 16.3 B

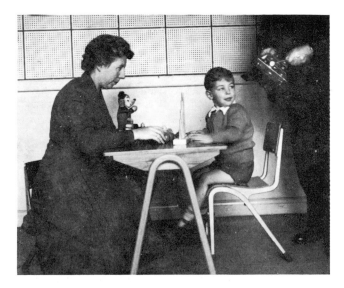

Fig. 16.3 C

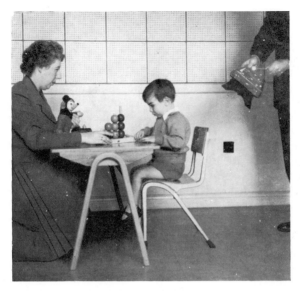

Fig. 16.3 D

Fig. 16.3   Hearing tests in children—the distraction technique (see text).

Once this exploratory stage is over, the child can be seated at a small table and distracted by the teacher or other observer (Figure 16.3, A). If severe deafness is present, a very loud sound may have to be used and, although it is open to many objections, the drum is useful for attracting attention (Figure 16.3, B). If he responds to the drum, a series of xylophone bars can be substituted and his reactions noted again (Figure 16.3, C). The examiner then moves further and further behind the child until there is no longer any response at all (Figure 16.3, D). Both drums and xylophone bars are capable of producing either faint or loud sounds; but these instruments should always be struck softly at first, because many of the children who are referred nowadays to audiology clinics may have no deafness at all. A variety of testing sounds will have to be used before one can gain a fairly accurate impression of the hearing capacity and no test of hearing can be regarded as complete until some attempt has been made to assess the child's reaction to the human voice.

Sound has so little meaning to the child who is born severely deaf that he will respond at first only to sounds which are well above his threshold intensity level, and it is not until he has been trained to use all his residual hearing that it is possible to assess his hearing loss with some accuracy.

In the first year or so of life, we must content ourselves with impressions, but at least we should be able to say whether a child has much hearing, little hearing or no hearing. And as he grows older, so does he become more and more responsive until, at about 3 or $3\frac{1}{2}$, he will begin to play more grown-up games.

Conditioning techniques

From the age of about 3 or $3\frac{1}{2}$ onwards, attempts can be made to 'condition' the child to carry out some simple act every time he hears a sound. The principle of these conditioning techniques can best be illustrated by a series of action shots taken during an actual test (Figure 16.4,).

The child is seated at a small table with a nest of coloured beakers. Opposite him sits the observer (in this case a teacher of the deaf) and beside her the examiner (Figure 16.4, A). The child is encouraged to look and to listen as a xylophone bar is struck and after the teacher has picked out the beakers two or three times, she holds the child's hand on the top remaining beaker and helps him to lift it out when he sees and hears the xylophone being struck again by the examiner (Figure 16.3, B). This is repeated as often as necessary until he appears to understand what is required of him. He is then allowed to do it himself (Figure 16.4, C). As soon as he has learnt this 'look and listen' game, the examiner goes behind him and the observer beckons him to listen (Figure 16.4, D). Every time he *hears* the sound, he will now pick out another cup and the examiner can go further and further away from him until he finds the greatest distance at which the child responds to this particular testing sound (Figure 16.4, E). Thereafter other frequencies and other sounds can be used.

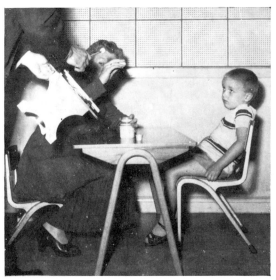

Fig. 16.4 A

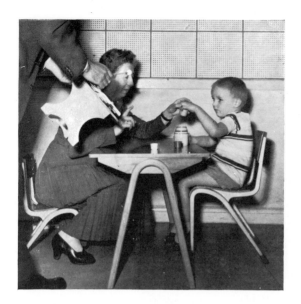

Fig. 16.4 B

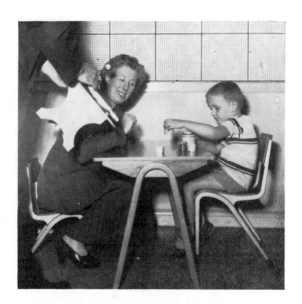

Fig. 16.4 C

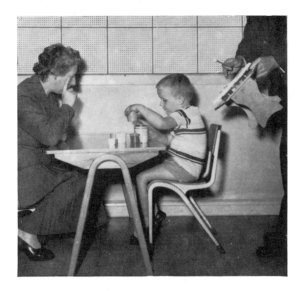

Fig. 16.4 D

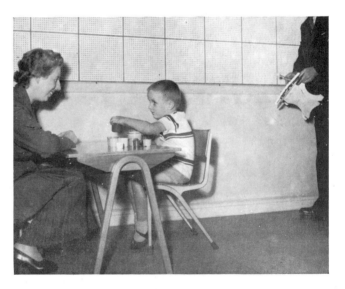

Fig. 16.4 E

Fig. 16.4   Hearing tests in children—the conditioning technique (see text).

In younger children, between 3 and $3\frac{1}{2}$, it may take several unhurried visits, perhaps of half an hour or more, before the conditioning response is fully established. It is always useful to start these tests with a drum or xylophone because the conditioning depends in the first place on looking as well as listening, and the movements of the hammer are easily seen. Sometimes the deaf child is so visually inclined that it may be difficult to persuade him not to look when the conditioning has been started with this 'look and listen' technique and it is then wiser to establish the response, from the beginning, from behind the child's back.

Once the response has been firmly established, however it is achieved, the test can be repeated with a wide variety of testing sounds—pitch pipes of different frequencies; the word 'Go'—this is often described as the 'Go' game; or any of the elements of speech —such as the high-pitched consonant sounds 's' and 'sh'. We can also use a small portable 'free-field' audiometer (see below), and the slightly older child can be conditioned to make the noise himself.

Audiometry in children

Soon after the child has been conditioned to the 'Go' game, he can be trained by similar play methods to respond to electrically-generated pure tones.

All the tests described above, both distracting and conditioning, are known as 'free field' tests because the testing sounds are made in a free field at some distance from the ears. Both ears are therefore tested at one and the same time and it is difficult or impossible to exclude (for example) a unilateral deafness by these methods. Furthermore, all the testing sounds so far mentioned are complex sounds and even the xylophone bars, carefully marked with their fundamental frequencies (500, 1000, 2000 and 4000 Hz) contain many overtones. And although our primary concern with children is to know how much or how little they hear of speech, no test of hearing is complete until we have also tested them with pure tones. The truth of this contention should be evident from the following case history.

A girl of 5, Gillian W., was referred to me with suspected deafness. Her mother had first had doubts about her hearing at the age of 2 because she was not talking. The mother's blood group was Rhesus-negative and Gillian was jaundiced at birth. Her tonsils and adenoids were removed at the age of 4, in the hope that she might have a simple 'catarrhal' deafness.

Her understanding of language was so poor that she could not be tested with word-pictures (which will be described below), but she was easily conditioned to the 'Go' game and was tested with xylophone bars of the frequencies 500, 1000, 2000 and 4000 Hz. She responded to each of these when they were struck very softly with a soft rubber hammer at a distance of 12 feet. She was then tested with unvoiced high-frequency consonant sounds delivered as softly as possible ('sh, 's', 'f', and 'th') and she showed a brisk conditioned response to all of them. Only when she was referred for a pure tone audiogram was it found that she had an abrupt loss of hearing in both ears above a frequency of 1000 Hz (Figure 16.5).

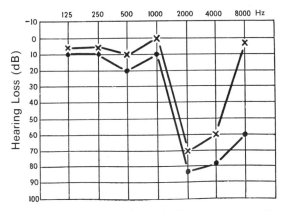

Fig. 16.5   Congenital high-tone deafness—pure tone audiogram.

If we were to accept the proposition that our *only* concern in testing a child's hearing is to determine the hearing for speech, this child at this particular stage would have passed the test. Yet she was a child of more than average ability, with no neurological signs but with defective speech and very poor language development, and her handicap was undoubtedly due, at least in part, to her hearing loss even though she responded readily to the softest high-pitched sounds of speech.

The tones of a pitch pipe are much purer (or less complex) than those of a xylophone bar and most of these cases of abrupt high-tone deafness will be detected by pitch pipes. But even these do not produce really pure tones and I am convinced that one cannot exclude deafness with absolute certainty until the hearing has been tested by pure tones. And since the pure tone audiogram is the only test at present which will give a true threshold response in each ear separately, it is to be favoured as an exclusory test.

The experienced technician can usually produce a reliable threshold response at about the age of 3 or $3\frac{1}{2}$. Occasionally there is some initial difficulty in persuading a child of this age to put on the headphones of the ordinary pure tone audiometer, and in 1947 Dix and Hallpike described their 'peep-show' audiometer in which no headphones had to be worn. Seated in front of the peep-show, the child was conditioned to press a button every time he heard a sound, and each time he pressed it a picture was lighted up. In more recent models, these pictures have been substituted by a changing kaleidoscope of coloured patterns.

But this is open to two chief objections: in the first place, it is much more expensive than the standard audiometer; in the second place, it is a 'free-field' audiometer in which both ears are tested together. It is therefore impossible to exclude a unilateral deafness and, in any event, there are few instances (if any) when the experienced technician cannot obtain an accurate threshold audiogram just as soon, with the added very distinct advantage that each ear can be tested separately.

Some characteristic audiograms from cases of congenital deafness will be discussed later (The Correlation of Cause and Effect) (page 154), but mention should perhaps be made before we leave this subject of a special conditioning technique described by Bordley and Hardy of Baltimore, in 1949. It has long been known that if a mild faradic (electric) shock was given to a child (or adult), there was increased sweating from the skin and that this was accompanied by changes in the electrical resistance in the skin. These changes in skin resistance can be recorded automatically on a roll of paper by an ink recording, and they formed the basis of Bordley and Hardy's Psycho-Galvanic Skin Resistance (P.G.S.R.) test. They found that if an auditory stimulus was given as a warning signal before such a shock, and if it was repeated several times, the child could be conditioned to give changes in the skin resistance every time the auditory stimulus was heard, in anticipation of the expected shock. A child thus conditioned to one tone would be conditioned also to any other tone that was audible to him, and it was claimed that an audiogram could be produced much earlier by this method than by any other. The results of this test are inconsistent and it has found little favour in this country.

It is of some historical importance but it has now been superceded by many other objective tests of hearing. (See page 54).

Voice and whisper tests

There are many ways in which the child's hearing for words or sentences can be tested by voice or whisper, and by far the best of them is the one devised by Michael Reed. This test is performed with phonetically balanced rhyming word-pictures—that is to say, the testing material consists of several series of monosyllabic rhyming words in picture form, with a carefully chosen selection of vowels and consonants (Figure 16.6). The top line, for example, shows the four rhyming words Door, Horse, Four and Ball, each with the same vowel sound ('aw') but each with different consonant sounds.

Before starting the test itself, it is important to go through all the pictures with the child to make certain that he can name them properly, and it need hardly be said that the test would lose some of its value if he called the horse a 'gee-gee', the ship a 'boat', or the feet 'toes'. When this has been done he is asked to point to the appropriate picture each time he hears the corresponding word. He is asked to 'show me the ball' or 'show me the fish'; 'the stool', 'the

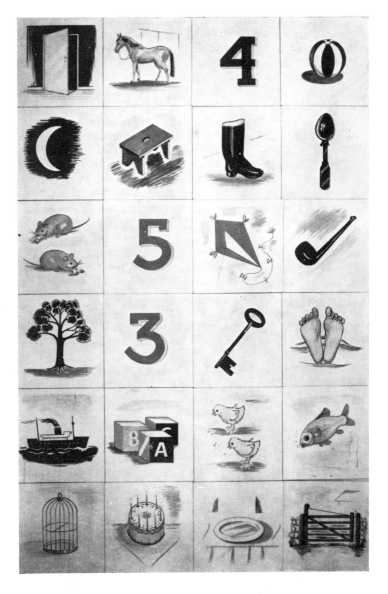

Fig. 16.6 Rhyming word-picture test (*M. Reed*).

mice', 'the gate'; 'tree', 'feet', 'three' and so on. And gradually the examiner moves further and further away from him until he has reached a distance of about 10 feet, or less if the child is confused.

The child who is able to distinguish all these words in a whispered voice at 6 feet or more almost certainly has normal hearing and the test is not open to the same fallacies as the conditioned response to the various elements of speech. The following case should demonstrate this point.

Jennifer J., a child of 8, was referred to me by a child psychiatrist. She was attending a school for severely maladjusted children and here it was noticed that 'her speech was poor'. To quote from the report, 'She tended to mishear words. It was thought, however, that this was a failure of discrimination rather than a hearing defect.' Her audiogram was almost identical with that of Gillian W. (see page 146). Similarly she gave reliable conditioned responses to the sounds 's', 'sh', 'f' and 'th', and also to the faint rustling of tissue paper, at a distance of 12 feet. Although these are all fundamentally high-frequency sounds, it was clear from her audiogram that she was not hearing anything above 1000 Hz, at this distance. But these are complex sounds and with normal hearing in the lower frequencies, she could respond to the lower-frequency components of the speech elements and the rustling paper. However, using the rhyming word-picture test, her deafness was quickly discovered. At 10 feet she could hear quite easily most of the words spoken in a soft conversational voice or even in a whisper, but she confused 'fish' with 'chick', and 'pipe' with 'kite' at 4 feet, and could not distinguish 'tree' from 'three' any further than 1 foot. It will be evident that when words are used for testing, it is not enough to be able to hear only *some* parts of the word; the child must be able to hear *every* part of *every* word to distinguish them with certainty. The most difficult pair of words appears to be the 'tree' and 'three', in which distinction is only possible if the child can hear the 'th' sound, the faintest of all the sounds of English speech and the one of highest frequency (see page 21).

This test is of particular value in detecting the presence or absence of partial deafness in children with defective speech and it can be repeated with a hearing aid, with lip-reading, or with both. It can be used in the average child from the age of 4 years onwards. In younger children, provided that they have some comprehension of speech, the test may be modified by using selected toys instead of pictures. This is an adaptation of Mary Sheridan's screening test, described below.

Screening tests of hearing in infants and young children. The diagnosis of congenital deafness is still established far too late far too often. How often does one hear the tragic story from the mother of a deaf child that she has taken her worst fears to her family doctor (or the otologist), only to be told that 'he'll be all right when he's a little older', or 'lots of children speak late', or 'nothing can be done till he's five, so don't worry'? Not uncommonly she has tried for months or even years to persuade her medical attendants that her child is deaf, before the chance meeting with another parent of a deaf child or the chance reading of some journalist's story brings her to some special clinic where facilities exist for the diagnosis and treatment of the handicap. It will take a long time to teach every practising doctor that congenital deafness can and should be diagnosed in the first year or so of life and that no child is too young to have his hearing examined. Until this happy state has been reached, some other method must be found of ensuring that every deaf child can have the best possible start in life. And this means early diagnosis.

It is to the great credit of Dr Berenice Humphreys, of Leicester, that she conceived the idea of screening the hearing of every child born in her own city within the first year life—clearly it would not be possible to diagnose every case of deafness at this age, because it is impossible to obtain a threshold response, but at least it should be possible to find those children who were severely deaf. In her capacity of Medical Officer to the Maternity and Child Welfare Department of a Local Health Authority, Dr Humphreys was in a position to see all the babies born in her own city. But this would be an impossible task for one person alone and so she thought that some of her Health Visitors could be trained to visit and screen the children in their homes or to see them in the clinics which they attended. The Health Visitor, after all had the unique advantage of visiting any child born in her own area and she was trained in general nursing and midwifery. She had also undertaken a special course of training which would equip her to visit the homes of young children. Furthermore the Health Visitor attended child welfare and other clinics for mothers and children and she already had training and experience in handling children and meeting their parents. But her primary function was that of a home visitor. So, argued Dr Humphreys, it might be possible to train a number of Health Visitors to carry out some relatively simple screening tests of hearing, although it was realized that not all of them would be suitable for this rather specialized type of work. The tests could be done in the clinic or the home.

Dr Humphreys took her ideas to the late Lady Ewing in Manchester and in 1952 a scheme was started in which the selected Health Visitors were trained to do these screening tests, under the supervision of Dr Humphreys, and in that year a special Audiology Clinic was set up in Leicester as part of the Child Welfare Service of the Local Authority.

In September 1957 Dr Humphreys published some of her results in the journal *Public Health*. Between June 1954 and May 1957, full screening tests had been given to 4409 children under the age of 5. Of this large number, only four were definitely found to be deaf and, of these four, there was a family history of deafness in no less than three. In only one picked up at 16 months, had there been no suspicion of deafness and no reason to expect it. There was a further very small number of children in whom deafness had not yet been excluded with certainty, but of the four established cases of deafness three were 'at risk because of the family history.

Theoretically at least, this finding of only one single unsuspected case of congenital deafness in over 4000 children would seem to be very little reward for such an enormous expenditure of time and effort, and it has been argued that such screening tests should be limited to those children who are known to be, for one reason or another, 'at risk'.

Which, then, are the vulnerable children? They include, in the first place, all children who have a family history of deafness; all children whose mothers have had rubella or other virus infections in the first three or four months of pregnancy; all babies who have had any birth injury, neonatal jaundice or anoxia; all children who were premature; and all children who may have *acquired* deafness in the early months or years of life, especially from meningitis or measles. Since a definite cause can be established in only about one-half of all cases of congenital deafness, we are still left with a large number of cases (the other half), who would escape undetected if we were to screen only those children with some known causative factor. We must therefore add two further groups of vulnerable children: those with cerebral palsy or other congenital abnormalities; and those who have a delay or defect in speech.

More recently Dr Irene Howarth, using a very similar list of vulnerable children, carried out an interesting controlled series of screening tests in Lancashire. First she examined 5531 children, from the general population, in 1955, 1956 and the first quarter of 1957. She found an incidence of deafness of 2·71 per 1000 children tested. During the last three quarters of 1957, she divided a further 3727 children into two groups—a vulnerable group and a control group. Of 662 vulnerable children tested the incidence of deafness per 1000 children was 9·06; of 3065 control children, the incidence was only 0·65—only two children in over three thousand. Hence the incidence of deafness was fourteen times greater in the vulnerable group than in the control group. These figures may appear to speak for themselves, but their interpretation has been challenged by Doctors Richards and Roberts, of the Department of Social and Occupational Medicine in the Welsh National School of Medicine. Their studies, published in 1967, led them to the conclusion that 'there is no alternative to the clinical examination of *all* infants in the neonatal period' (my italics), and there is growing agreement that all children should be screened between the ages of seven and nine months, and again shortly after entering school.

In all screening tests, as opposed to diagnostic tests, one starts with the assumption that the hearing is probably normal and it cannot be too strongly emphasized that their main function is to detect all those children who have *normal* hearing. Every child who fails to produce normal responses must be referred as soon as possible to a specialized clinic, where the cause of failure will be determined. It is customary to use faint sounds to which the normal child is likely to respond, but the choice of the actual method will depend, of course, on the age of the child, and there are at least two age-groups in which these tests should be carried out: some time during the first year of life; and as soon as possible after entry to school at the age of 5. In addition, the hearing should be screened, at the school medical inspections, in any child whose progress stops suddenly.

The 'first year' test

All children should be examined within the first year of life and some Local Health Authorities in this country have introduced a 'Birthday Examination' at about the time of every child's first birthday. It is not suggested that the screening tests of hearing (or of sight) should be carried out as isolated tests, but rather that they should be incorporated, when they are indicated, within the framework of this general examination.

The normal infant is most easily tested between the 7th and 9th months, when it is a relatively simple matter to examine him with the distraction techniques described above (see 'Diagnostic Tests of Hearing in Infants and Young Children'). The sounds used should be faint sounds but it is also important that they should be *meaningful* sounds. Many a child at this age will pay little or no attention to the banging of a drum or the clapping of hands, but he will nearly always react briskly to the much fainter sounds which have meaning to him in his everyday activities—the soft call of his name in his mother's voice; the squeaking of a favourite toy; the sound of his rattle; or the clinking of a spoon on a cup, especially if he is bottle fed. There is also a strange but unfailing fascination at this age for the crinkling of tissue paper. All these sounds are complex sounds, and at this age infants react much more readily to complex than to pure tones.

Dr Mary Sheridan has examined the hearing of many hundreds of normal hearing children, and she has described a comprehensive and beautifully standardized set of screening tests for use with children of different ages. (The Stycar test.)

The child, seated on his mother's lap, is distracted by an observer and the test can be started as soon as he has settled down. Each ear should be tested separately from a distance of 3 feet or more, and the examiner should stand to each side of the child, just outside his range of vision. The normal reaction of the hearing child is a brisk turning of the head but he will often show no response at all if the sound is made immediately behind him or immediately above his head. One of the most convincing reactions I have seen was made by a baby boy only 10 weeks old who was brought into the clinic half-asleep in his mother's arms. He had been bottle fed from birth and the faintest clinking of a spoon on the edge of a cup at a distance of 10 feet brought forth an instantaneous sucking movement of the tongue and lips.

These simple distraction tests will certainly pick out children with severe degrees of hearing loss and, if they are properly performed by a skilled examiner, will also bring to light some of the slighter degrees of partial deafness in many other children. But by scientific standards these are relatively crude tests and some children (especially those with high-tone deafness) will pass through the screen at this age. It is therefore necessary to have a further check at some later stage, and it is convenient to do this when the child goes to school, provided of course that there has been no reason to suspect deafness in the meantime.

The primary 'school entry' test

As soon as possible after the age of 5, every school entrant should have a further screening test. This serves to pick out those children who have passed through the coarser mesh of the earlier screen; it will also pick up those who have acquired deafness in the intervening years, or those who suffer from a progressive deafness of congenital origin.

The method most widely used is the 'sweep frequency' test described by the Ewings. Using a pure tone audiometer, the examiner (usually the School Sister) 'sweeps' through a limited range of frequencies in octave or half-octave steps at a fixed intensity level of 15 or 20 decibels. The frequencies chosen are the so-called speech frequencies and although six frequencies have been used, four should probably be enough—500, 1000, 2000 and 4000 Hz. The test is first explained to a group of children, about twenty or twenty-five at a time, but each child is examined separately. He is asked to indicate whether or not he hears each of the testing tones in each ear separately, and if he does he passes the test. It is assumed, in choosing an intensity of 15 or 20 dB, that the child who can hear the speech frequencies at this level will not be handicapped educationally. But this point has yet to be proved.

The 'sweep frequency' test can be performed by an experienced operator at the rate of one child every three minutes, but it is a pure-tone test and does not tell us anything about the child's understanding for speech. It should therefore be combined with another 'voice and whisper' test, and the rhyming word-picture test of Michael Reed (page 147) deserves a much wider application as a screening test for school entrants. The words should be spoken in a whispered voice at a distance of 6 feet and the child will pass the test if he can hear and understand all the words in each ear at this distance.

Either of these screening tests—the 'First Year' test or the Primary 'School Entry' test—can, of course, be modified for use as full diagnostic tests. But skill is not easily won in testing small children, and it must be realized that they are in fact only screening tests and nothing but screening tests. Providing their limitations are recognized, they can be of inestimable value in picking up the deaf child much earlier than would otherwise be the case.

The secondary 'school entry' test

It is now statutory in some areas to screen the hearing of children again just before or just after entry to the Secondary Schools, at about the age of 12 years. Although many of them will not be deaf, any child who fails these screening tests should be referred without delay for full diagnostic tests of hearing to a special Audiology Unit or Clinic where facilities exist for this sort of work. If this rule were applied also to every child whose parents have suspected deafness, there would be very few of the tragedies that one sees almost daily in working with these unfortunate children.

The correlation of cause and effect. In July 1955, L. Fisch reported the results of an investigation in which he had tried to correlate the type and degree of deafness with its cause.

Although we are always concerned with a child's hearing for speech, the pure tone audiogram is the only reliable 'threshold' test of hearing and the only one which gives us a well-defined 'pattern' of the hearing loss. There has been no large-scale investigation into the correlation of audiograms with the other tests of hearing in children, but Fisch studied a group of 250 cases of congenital deafness in which a reliable pure tone audiogram was available and the cause of the deafness had been established.

Since there are several different pathologies of *hereditary* deafness, it is not surprising that there were several different types of audiometric pattern in children whose deafness had been caused by genetic weakness. It may be 'flat', with an equal or near-equal hearing loss at all frequencies (Figure 16.7, A); or 'sloping', with a greater loss for high tones than for low tones (Figure 16.7, B) or, much less commonly, with a greater loss for low tones than for high tones (Figure 16.7, C). It is interesting that several cases of the Waardenburg syndrome have shown this last type of audiogram. Occasionally, there are only 'islands' of hearing in the lowest frequencies (Figure 16.7D) and in these cases the response is probably to vibration rather than to true hearing as we normally understand it. This type of audiogram may therefore be produced by those who are born totally deaf. Although there is such a wide range of audiometric patterns in cases of hereditary congenital deafness, there tends to be one particular pattern for any one particular family.

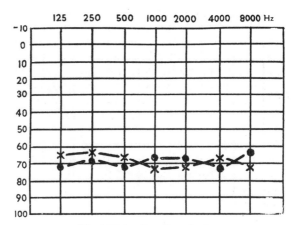

Fig. 16.7 A.   Heredity—flat 'curve .

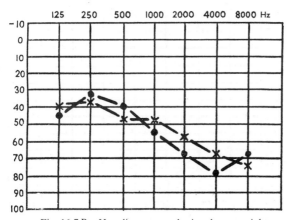

Fig. 16.7 B.   Heredity—curve sloping down to right.

Fig. 16.7   Congenital deafness—correlation of cause and effect. (*L. Fisch.*) (Pure tone audiograms.)

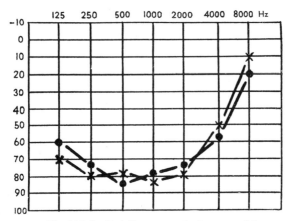

Fig. 16.7 C.   Heredity—curve sloping up to right.

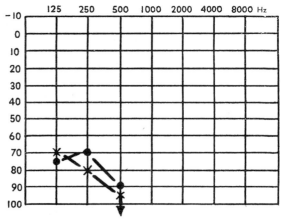

Fig. 16.7 D.   Heredity—'islands' of low tone hearing.

Fig. 16.7   (Pure tone audiograms *contd.*)

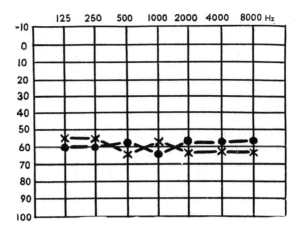

Fig. 16.7 E.   Pre-natal group—flat 'curve'.

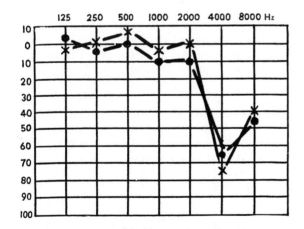

Fig. 16.7 F.   Perinatal group—abrupt high tone loss.

Fig. 16.7   (Pure tone audiograms *contd.*)

In congenital deafness due to maternal rubella or other pre-natal causes, the lesion is in the cochlea and there is a general arrest in development of the organ of Corti. And since there is a uniform under-development of the organ as a whole, there is a more or less uniform loss of hearing over the whole frequency range. This produces a characteristic 'flat' audiogram, commonly at a level of about 60 dB (Figure 16.7, E).

On the other hand, the most typical feature of the perinatal group is a selective hearing loss for the high tones (Figure 16.7, F).

Why should this be so?

It has already been said that in this group the lesion is in the cochlear nuclei. There are two cochlear nuclei on each side of the brain-stem, one 'dorsal' and one 'ventral', and there is in these nuclei a sharp separation of the high tones and the low tones. The nerve fibres which carry high tones are concentrated in the dorsal nucleus and it is in this nucleus that the lesion mainly occurs in kernicterus and anoxia.

Can this be explained?

Fisch believes that there is probably a combination of circum-stances. In the first place, that part of the auditory apparatus which is responsible for hearing the higher frequencies is much younger than the rest, in terms of development of the species; and it is known that the younger the cells are, in the development of a species, the more vulnerable they are to noxious influences. They are therefore the first cells to be affected in any destructive process. Secondly, the dorsal cochlear nucleus is more exposed than the ventral one. And thirdly, the dorsal nucleus has an unusually rich supply of capillary blood vessels which demands a greater consumption of oxygen. It is therefore more susceptible to oxygen lack (anoxia). He goes on to say that the amount of damage done by these perinatal influences is proportionate to the extent of the pathological change. A slight degree of damage will affect only the dorsal cochlear nucleus, leading to an abrupt and selective high-tone loss; a severer degree will affect a part of the ventral nucleus also, producing a marked high-tone loss with some loss for low tones as well; and when the pathological changes are very great, the widespread damage will often produce mental deficiency or other neurological complications which may 'mask' any deafness that is present. In extreme cases they will be incompatible with survival, and it is possibly for this reason that only the 'high-tone' type of audiogram is seen in these cases.

There is no absolute or constant relationship between cause and effect but one *can* say, broadly speaking, that the hereditary group can cause damage of any type and any degree, and that any audio-metric pattern is possible; that the pre-natal group usually damages the organ of Corti uniformly throughout its whole length, thus producing a flat audiogram; and that the perinatal group commonly damages the cochlear nuclei (first and foremost the dorsal nucleus), with a characteristic high-tone loss.

Further work along these lines may, in the future, give us much-needed help in establishing the pathology, if not always the cause, of congenital deafness, in some of those many cases which must still be recorded as 'cause unknown'.

The differential diagnosis of congenital deafness. There are several conditions which may be confused with congenital deafness and these will be discussed separately.

Deafness acquired in early childhood

If deafness is acquired during the early years of life, its effects on speech and language are very similar to those of congenital deafness. Particularly does this apply to the first two years, but profound deafness may cause serious effects on speech and language even when it is acquired as late as seven or eight.

The commonest causes of severe sensori-neural deafness in early childhood are the acute febrile illnesses, especially the three M's: measles, mumps, and meningitis (see page 186).

Deafness in childhood is sometimes attributed to head injuries, and simple 'catarrhal' deafness must not be forgotten.

Innate intellectual inferiority

It has been said that any child who is not talking by the age of 2 is probably deaf or backward, and indeed it used to be a common fallacy that most deaf children were themselves backward. But it is now known that the range of intelligence levels in deaf children is the same as that in hearing children and that the *average* deaf child has the same innate ability as the *average* hearing one.

The distinction between deafness and backwardness can only be made correctly if the right tests are used, and ideally the intelligence of deaf children should be assessed only by those who are accustomed to dealing with them and are familiar with their problems. Verbal tests demand normal hearing, and their indiscriminate application to the deaf child will inevitably give him too low a score. I have heard of the case of a girl in a special school for partially hearing children who had had her intelligence assessed on two separate occasions at yearly intervals and on each occasion she had been reported to be Educationally Sub-Normal (ESN). In spite of the examiner's low estimate of her ability, her teacher was convinced, by her general response to learning, that she was of at least average intelligence. When the girl was summoned for her third annual examination, the teacher asked that she might be present. Again, for the third time, she was assessed as Educationally Sub-Normal. Referring back to one particular test item, the teacher asked the examiner how he had marked it.

'Oh, she failed that one,' said the examiner. 'When I asked her to draw a diamond, she drew one; but when I asked her to draw it bigger, she just drew a *squiggle*.'

'Are you going to accept that?' asked the teacher. 'Are you sure she *heard* you?'

'She must have heard me,' assured the examiner, 'or she wouldn't have drawn anything.'

'Yes, she must have heard *something*,' said the teacher, 'but do you know *what* she heard?' Then, turning to the girl and pointing to the squiggle, 'Sonia, what did the man say to you when you did that?'

'Draw a *squiggle*,' replied the girl.

The partially deaf child can easily confuse the words 'bigger' and 'squiggle', each with the same vowel sounds and each with the same cadences—which was all that this girl *heard*.

It is clearly pointless to test the intelligence of a deaf or partially hearing child with verbal tests, for these demand an understanding of the spoken word. Performance tests (such as the Merrill-Palmer and Wechsler tests) should always be used, and indeed this should also apply to any child who is not known to have normal hearing. It is, in fact, probably wise to test the intelligence of all children with both verbal and performance tests (as in the Wechsler tests), when any discrepancy in favour of the performance items will suggest the likelihood of deafness.

From time to time, partially hearing children of average intelligence were sent to ESN Schools simply because the wrong sort of test had been used. Usually these children were found to have a high-tone deafness.

Much more serious is the group of deaf children who spend their lives in institutions for mental defectives. Neurotic reactions may be common among deaf children as a result of their deafness and consequent frustration, and it may be very difficult sometimes to decide whether children who have acquired no speech are deaf, mentally defective, or emotionally disturbed; or whether they are suffering from a combination of these conditions. Only prolonged observation will solve the riddle, and in March 1953 a research unit was established at the Belmont Hospital in Sutton (Surrey) for the study of apparently deaf children with defective speech, and behaviour problems. Three years later, Dawson and her colleagues (Miss Evans, a teacher of the deaf; Michael Reed, an educational psychologist; and Dr Louis Minski, a psychiatrist) recorded their findings in the *Journal of Mental Science*. They found that 'some children who have never spoken and who are therefore inaccessible and who may be asocial or antisocial in their behaviour are diagnosed as being mentally defective and spend their lives in mentally defective institutions'. A number of these children proved to be deaf. Thanks to improved diagnostic methods, this sort of misplacement is very rare today.

'Congenital auditory impreception'
There is a group of children who hear but do not understand. And because they do not understand, they do not speak. Their hearing as tested by audiometry or by simple conditioning techniques, is normal; but their understanding, as evidenced by their failure to recognize their own names or to carry out simple commands, is at fault. Speech and language have no meaning to them.

This condition is a form of sensory, or receptive, or auditory, 'aphasia'—that is to say, there is some fault in the sensory nervous pathways for speech. To it is given the title 'Congenital Word-Deafness' or 'Congenital Auditory Imperception'. In 1930 Professor Sir Alexander Ewing examined ten children who were reported to have congenital imperception and no fewer than six of them had high-tone deafness; and it must be remembered that the deaf child may also be aphasic.

In the absence of pathological studies the site of the lesion must remain pure conjecture. Theoretically, it should be central; it should be bilateral; and it may be in the 'psycho-auditory' area (see page 24).

Deprivation
Some children fail to talk at the usual age simply through lack of opportunity to learn. The baby who spends all the time between his feeds tucked away in his pram at the bottom of a garden cannot be expected to speak as early as the one whose mother talks to him throughout his waking hours. He is deprived of the experience of listening. There is also evidence that children who are exposed to an environment of mixed languages tend sometimes to be later in talking than those whose parents both speak the mother tongue.

Family delay in speech
When all the known causes have been excluded, there still remains yet another group of children whose speech is delayed, and in some of these one hears the story that 'his father didn't speak till he was three' or, 'none of his sisters spoke till they were four'.

This should be the very last diagnosis, if indeed it should ever be made, and much further research is needed to elucidate this and many other problems of the late talker.

The classification of deafness in children

There is no really satisfactory classification of deafness in children, as there are so many 'variables'.

We can classify it according to *type* and distinguish congenital deafness from acquired deafness, conductive deafness from sensori-neural deafness. Or we can define the hearing-loss, according to the audiogram, as a 'flat' loss, or a 'high-tone' loss, or a 'low-tone' loss.

We can classify it according to *degree* and we can fix an arbitrary dividing line between a total or sub-total deafness on the one hand, and a partial deafness on the other. And we can further subdivide partial deafness into secondary degrees of 'slight', or 'moderate', or 'severe'. But here certain difficulties arise. For example, the child who hears normally (on the audiogram) at 500 and 1000 Hz but has an abrupt drop to 80 dB at 2000 and 4000 Hz will have an *average* hearing loss of 40 dB for the so-called 'speech frequencies'. Yet in most instances, his handicap will almost certainly be less severe than that of a child who has a 'flat' loss of 40 dB at each of these frequencies, although the 'average' hearing loss is the same in both. Moreover, the steady advance in the development of electronic equipment must surely change our conception of which children we regard as 'deaf' and which as 'partially deaf'. And many a child who was regarded (and educated) as a 'deaf' child 20 or 25 years ago must now, with modern aids to hearing, be regarded (and educated) as a 'partially' deaf child, in so far as he can be expected to acquire speech and language by these *un*-natural means.

The last serious attempt to classify deaf children depended very largely on the presence or absence of *naturally*-acquired speech and language, when a Special Committee of the Board of Education, in 1938, issued their 'Report on Children with Defective Hearing'. According to this report, the 'Deaf' (or Grade III) child was one whose hearing was so defective and whose speech and language were so little developed that he required education by methods used for deaf children *without naturally-acquired speech or language*. The 'Partially Deaf' (or Grade II) child was one whose hearing was so defective that he required for his education special arrangements, or facilities, but not the educational methods used for 'deaf' children without naturally-acquired speech or language. The Grade I child was one who, despite defective hearing, could nevertheless obtain proper benefit from the education provided in an ordinary school without any special arrangements of any kind.

At the time of writing, the 1938 Report is almost forty years out of date. When all is said and done, we want to know as many facts as possible about each child before we begin to classify him: when his deafness was detected; whether it is congenital or acquired; whether it is conductive or sensori-neural; whether his hearing loss affects all tones equally or some more than others; what is his hearing for speech; what his own speech is like, and what his development of language; how he communicates with others, and others with him; whether he has any other handicap; what of his innate ability; and what of his home background and the attitude of his parents. Only when we know all these and any other relevant details can we begin to understand his problems. But every child is an individual, not to be dominated by any hard-and-fast set of rules, and even when we know all the facts, our ultimate decisions about him must still depend on the personal conscience, the personal experience and the personal philosophy of each and every individual who is entrusted with his present and his future.

The educational treatment of deafness in children

The vast majority of children who are born deaf have a sensori-neural deafness, as also do many others who have acquired deafness (as from meningitis) early in childhood. Unfortunately it is true to say that no treatment, either medical or surgical, is of any avail in these cases, and their management depends entirely on educational methods. Some of these methods can and should be applied also to children suffering from conductive deafness who, by virtue of their handicap, are retarded educationally.

It is perhaps unfortunate that the word 'Deafness' is used to cover such a wide degree of hearing defects, but it is used here to indicate any defect of hearing, whether total or partial, congenital or acquired, conductive or sensori-neural. And I believe that it is only in this context that one can review the educational treatment of deafness as a whole.

Historical note on the education of deaf children. Forty five years ago, C. Shaw, then Assistant Inspector of Special Schools (Blind and Deaf) to the London County Council, wrote an article on the Education and Welfare of the Deaf and Dumb in the fourteenth edition of the *Encyclopaedia Britannica.* He records that 'in the early ages the deaf were regarded as idiots and were killed out of hand. They had no place in the order of things and were regarded as mere encumbrances.'

'Up to nearly the end of the nineteenth century,' he adds, 'the education of the deaf was provided for mostly by charity.'

What sort of education was this?

The late R. Scott Stevenson, one time Chairman of the National Institute for the Deaf and an old chief of mine, tells us (in the *History of Otolaryngology,* written with the late Douglas Guthrie) that 'The Venerable Bede (born about A.D. 673) speaks of a dumb youth being taught by St John of Beverley, to repeat letters and syllables and then words and sentences, but at the time this was regarded as a miracle'.

'It was in Spain in the sixteenth century,' he continues, 'that the systematic education of the deaf and dumb was begun for religious motives, by a Benedictine monk, Pedro Ponce de Leon. . . .' His writings have been lost, but his work was continued by another Benedictine monk, Juan Pablo Bonet, whose book contained a manual alphabet almost identical with that in use today in Europe and America; nevertheless his method of teaching—and he had a number of pupils—was *oral.* That is to say, he taught the deaf to speak. Bonet published a monograph on the *Art of Teaching the Deaf to Speak* in 1620 and Sir Kenelm Digby, mentioning it in his *Treatise Concerning Bodies* in 1644, describes how a Spanish lord, born deaf, was taught to speak by a priest. 'He could not govern the pitch of his voice,' he says; 'what he delivered he ended in the same key as he began it.' Digby also noted that he studied attentively the face of anyone who spoke to him, and that he could interpret nothing in the dark.

The first person in Britain to devote himself to the education of the deaf was one John Bulwer who, in 1644, published his *Chironomia, or the Art of Manual Rhetorique.* He dealt with gesture as a natural means of communication in Man, but there was no attempt to construct a manual alphabet. Indeed, he also was an 'oralist' and four years later he published another book called *Philocophus or the Deafe and Dumbe Man's Friend,* in which he claimed that 'a man born deaf and dumb may be taught to heare the sound of words with his eye, and thence learn to speake with his tongue'. This lip-reading he called 'Ocular Audition'.

The 'oral' method continued both in this country and abroad, and in 1692 Dr Jan Amman, a Swiss physician who practised in Holland, published his book *Surdus Loquens* (or 'the Talking Deaf Man'). He insisted on the importance of a purely 'oral' method of teaching and his book laid the foundations of the one now so widely practised and approved. But the Abbé Charles de l'Epée (1712–89) made an entirely new departure from the established practice of this time when he developed the signs used naturally by the deaf into a systematic and conventional sign-language.

The first School for the Deaf and Dumb in Britain was set up at Edinburgh in 1760 by Thomas Braidwood. In that year a deaf-mute boy was sent to Braidwood's school—then an ordinary school—to learn to write, and within a few years he had taught the boy not only to write but also to speak. After this success, he devoted himself to teaching the deaf, and Scott Stevenson recalls that 'Braidwood's school was visited by Dr Samuel Johnson and his biographer James Boswell'. Writing of this visit in his *Journey to the Western Islands of Scotland,* Dr Johnson says: 'The improvement of Mr Braidwood's pupils is wonderful. They not only speak, write and understand what is written but if he that speaks looks towards them and modifies his organ by distinct and full utterance, they know so well what is spoken, that it is an expression scarcely figurative to say that they hear with the eye. . . . It was pleasing to see one of the most desperate of human calamities capable of so much help; whatever enlarges hope, will exalt courage; after having seen the deaf taught arithmetick, who would be afraid to cultivate the Hebrides?'

Braidwood kept his method secret, but it was thought to be a combination of lip-reading and signs—of oralism and manualism.

Braidwood moved his school to London in 1783, when he established it at Grove House, Mare Street, Hackney. There he died in 1806, at the age of 90, and the school was continued after his death by his daughter and two grandsons. In 1792, the London Asylum for the Deaf and Dumb was set up in the Old Kent Road (Fig. 16.8), and its first principal was a nephew and former assistant of Thomas Braidwood's, one Dr Joseph Watson.

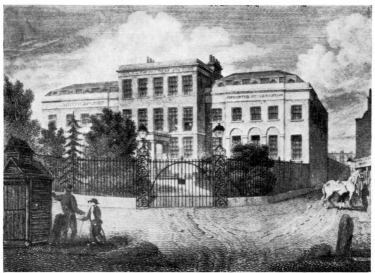

Fig. 16.8   The Deaf and Dumb Asylum, Kent Road. This is a photograph of a print, dated 1816, in the author's possession. The 'asylum' is now the Old Kent Road School for the Deaf, one of the junior schools for deaf children administered by the Greater London Council.

Denmark was the first country to introduce the *compulsory* education of deaf children, in 1817, and it was not until 1893 that the report of the Royal Commission which had been appointed to consider the condition of the blind and deaf in Britain, was published. As a result, the Elementary Education (Blind and Deaf Children) Act was passed, and it provided for the compulsory attendance at school of deaf children between 7 and 16 years of age. In 1937, the compulsory age for attendance of deaf children in schools was reduced from 7 to 5, and the Education Act of 1946 ensured that they could be accepted for admission from the age of 2 years if the parents so desired.

In 1884, a College of Teachers of the Deaf was founded. This is now the National College of Teachers of the Deaf, which grants a special Diploma approved by the Department of Education and Science.

The University of Manchester opened a special department for the training of teachers of the deaf in 1919. This is now the Department of Audiology and Education of the Deaf, under the direction of Professor Ian Taylor. Another similar department was started in London, at the Institute of Education, in 1965; and there are also new departments at Oxford and Edinburgh.

David Wright, a distinguished poet, gives a detailed historical account of the education of the deaf in his fascinating autobiography,

Deafness: A Personal Account.

Manualism. The Latin word *manus* means 'a hand' and the term 'manualism' can be applied to any method which teaches people to communicate by hand. This may range from simple gesture, through finger-spelling, to a fully developed sign-language. We all use gesture to some extent—though the staid Britisher usually reserves it for moments of emotional crisis—and my friend Dr Pierre Gorman, himself born deaf, has written that 'a difficulty facing the deaf person in the English culture is its insistence that normal persons, when speaking, should communicate with a minimum of facial and bodily gestures. This robs the deaf person of many valuable visible cues in conversation and makes it much more difficult than it would be on the Continent, where such gestures form a natural feature of the conversation between normal persons.'

There are several forms of manual communication: *sign language* is used mainly by people who have been born deaf, and the signs are based on ideas or pictures, rather than on words; in *finger spelling*, a visible symbol is used to represent each letter of the alphabet and words are simply spelt out letter by letter; *cued speech* gives manual indications of the sounds of speech. Unlike finger-spelling, it is based on phonetics and may therefore reinforce lip-reading and speech; the *Danish mouth-hand system* is also phonetic and is used in conjunction with lip-reading. Only the consonant sounds are indicated by the hand; and the *Paget-Gorman systematic sign system* is a grammatical form of signing in which each word is indicated.

'Manualism' must have been used, to a greater or lesser extent, for as long as the deaf have come together, and one has only to visit a school for the deaf—out of class hours—or a club or mission for the deaf, to realize that it is the 'natural' language of the gregarious deaf. Moreover the gregarious deaf are the segregated deaf, and if the deaf are to be integrated into normal society they must be taught to communicate by word of mouth. It may have a useful role, not only in providing an earlier introduction to language for some handicapped children, but also as a reinforcement for other methods of communication; but the limitations of any sign language lie in its lack of speed and in the narrow cultural context in which it can develop. 'Oralism', or the method of training the deaf to communicate (literally) 'by word of mouth', has now largely replaced the manual method (officially) in nearly all of the Schools for the Deaf and the Partially

Hearing in Great Britain.

Oralism. The culminating point in the movement towards 'oralism' came at the International Congress of Teachers of the Deaf at Milan, in 1880, when the delegates decided by a large majority that the oral system provided the best means of educating *most* deaf children. As Scott Stevenson put it in his second book of reminiscences (*Goodbye, Harley Street*): 'It was at the International Congress . . . at Milan . . . that amid scenes of great enthusiasm all methods of educating the deaf other than the oral system were flung out of the window'.

If it be accepted—and it is accepted by *most* of our teachers of the deaf today—that *most* deaf children can be taught to communicate by speech, then oralism is the order of the day. But this is a two-way system wherein the deaf child must not only be taught to understand the speech of others but must also be taught to speak in such a way that others can understand him. And his understanding of speech must derive from all the senses, or parts of them, which remain to him.

Lip-reading

It is common knowledge that a child who is deprived of one or other of his senses will very often cultivate the others to his own great advantage. And mention has already been made of the child born partially deaf who is 'all eyes'. The term 'partially deaf' is used advisedly in this context, for very few (if any) children who are born totally deaf appear to develop this *natural* facility for lip-reading. It would seem that the presence of at least *some* residual hearing, however slight, is an essential stimulus to the search for visual clues; in other words, the child born deaf must have enough hearing to make him aware that speech or language exists before he begins to *look* for what he *cannot hear*. And whatever hearing he may have, the early use of a hearing aid will promote his natural (as opposed to his un-natural, or taught) development of lip-reading.

There is a group of children, including some with very severe degrees of partial deafness, who appear to be born with that 'natural aptitude for visual communication' (Wendy Galbraith) which incites them to develop, quite spontaneously, a truly remarkable facility for lip-reading. These are the children who 'get by', who 'hold their own' in a normal hearing environment for many months and sometimes many years before the true nature of their handicap is discovered by the demonstration of a hearing defect, often unexpectedly severe. This may be related, in some way not yet fully determined, to a superior intelligence; but it can certainly occur also in children of only average ability or less. The problem awaits solution, but it is one that must be solved because it may have a very significant bearing on the type of deaf child (or more correctly, the type of partially hearing child) who is likely to benefit from education in a normal hearing environment. And if this rather indeterminate 'aptitude' could be assessed at an early age, one could avoid many of the subsequent frustrations that may result from the sense of failure in a too-deaf child in a hearing environment.

It is probable that every individual, whether hearing or deaf, falls into one or other of two groups: one with a particularly good 'visual', and one with a better innate 'auditory', aptitude. And there is going on at present, in Denmark, an investigation into the visual and auditory abilities inherent in hearing people.

A number of children have so little hearing that they can be taught to communicate by speech only through what they see and what they feel is very small.

Auditory training

The majority of deaf children, however, whether their deafness be congenital or acquired, have some residual hearing; and in many (perhaps in most) instances this can and should be trained.

There is nothing new in the idea of 'auditory training' for it has been known for many, many years that many children born deaf could be taught to speak, albeit imperfectly, if their mothers spoke to them often enough and loud enough. But auditory training really came into its own with the introduction of the hearing aid, and particularly the individual aid which could be worn by the child all day. And there have been constant and dramatic improvements in the design and performance of these instruments over the last twenty-five years or so.

Until only thirty-five years or so ago, children had to content themselves with group aids, whose use was confined to the special schools because individual aids were far too heavy. At home, all (or most) was silent. But with the inception of the National Health Service, came an aid that could be obtained free of charge by every deaf child (or adult) in Britain. A very big one it was, too; but it has become smaller and smaller and the current model compares favourably, in size at least, with many commercial aids; and more powerful commercial aids, both body-worn and head-worn, are available to those children who need them, on the recommendation of an otologist.

The modern electronics engineer has produced a wide range of acoustic equipment which brings sound within the reach of most deaf children. Furthermore, there has been some considerable improvement recently in 'matching' the frequency response of an aid to the type of hearing loss, as assessed with the audiometer. But this does not mean that all of those who can hear sound will necessarily hear and understand *speech*—or even parts of speech. And it is only after training all of a child's residual hearing, probably for at least a year, that one can say whether this child should use an aid, or that child should not.

Professor Sir Alexander Ewing, in his *Educational Guidance and the Deaf Child,* said that although a child's *hearing for speech* may not be helped much by an aid when his hearing loss exceeds 80 decibels, he may, nevertheless, be able 'to follow speech more accurately and more quickly when using the aid to supplement lip-reading than by lip-reading alone' even with hearing losses as great as 95 decibels. But the ability of an individual child to derive benefit from a hearing aid depends, not only on the extent of his hearing loss, but also on the age at which his handicap is ascertained, on the cause of his deafness and on many other factors besides – especially on the amount and quality of the auditory training which he receives; and the quantity and quality of the training received by many of these children still leave much to be desired.

Furthermore, some children learn more easily from 'aural' impressions, others from 'visual' impressions; some of us can assimilate more knowledge from a lecture than from a book, others the reverse. And there can be no doubt that some deaf children with very severe hearing losses can gain much more from auditory training than others with much less severe losses. It may be that these are the 'aural' children.

But if modern acoustic equipment is so powerful and its frequency responses so wide, why should auditory training be necessary? Reference to speech audiograms provides at least part of the answer. Any child (or adult) who has a sensori-neural deafness can be helped (theoretically) to some degree by making speech louder. Beyond a certain critical point, however, further amplification will contrive to make speech louder, but its intelligibility diminishes. The sounds of speech are distorted. Now, the child who is born deaf has no preformed 'patterns' of speech in the central parts of his auditory nervous pathway and his speech centres can be trained to distinguish the new, distorted patterns which reach them through the aid. They do not hear the words as we hear them, but they can be taught that a certain sound which we hear as 'boat', and which they may hear (for example) as 'bow', may represent either 'boat' or 'bowl' or 'bow'. And blessed with enough hearing, they can with further training learn to distinguish the one from the others, often by hearing alone. This 'auditory discrimination', as it is called, is a hardwon prize which must be cherished and nurtured throughout his life.

Wendy Galbraith has devised a 'pyramid' of the stages in auditory training (Figure 16.9) which lead finally to full *speech discrimination,* these stages being affected by (amongst other things) the age of the child; the degree of his hearing loss; previous experience; the child's attitude to his hearing aid; opportunity; and intelligence.

There are, of course, limitations to auditory training. Not all children (or adults, either) are capable of reaching the top of the 'pyramid', and it goes without saying that no child who is totally deaf can be 'auditorily' trained. But electronic equipment is now

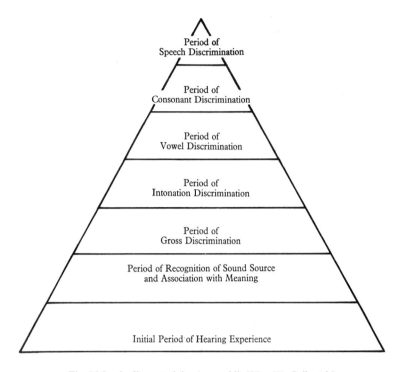

Fig. 16.9 Auditory training 'pyramid'. (*Miss W. Galbraith.*)

more powerful than it was ten or fifteen years ago, *much* more so than it was twenty or twenty-five years ago, and many a child can now benefit from auditory training who only a decade ago would have been regarded (quite rightly) as beyond its help.

But here, perhaps, it may be opportune to issue a warning. There is some evidence that, in rather rare instances, the residual hearing may be actually damaged by the extremely powerful instruments which are now available, and all of those who are responsible for prescribing aids to severely deaf children should keep a very careful check on the hearing, preferably by serial audiograms, of those children to whom these very powerful aids have been issued—especially as there is a growing tendency to recommend the simultaneous use of aids in both ears together. (Binaural listening, with the use of two complete hearing aids, may improve both sound localization and speech discrimination). Should there be any sign at all of deterioration in the hearing, it is prudent to remove the aid from one ear, at least until such time as it becomes certain whether this deterioration is within the natural history of the causative lesion, or whether it may be due to 'acoustic trauma'.

Methods of training must be adapted to advances, as and when they occur, and we must be prepared to change our conceptions of 'deafness' and 'partial deafness' (or 'partial hearing') as each new one appears.

Educational techniques must therefore be flexible and we must try to resist the all-too-common temptation to 'pigeon-hole' each child into a rigid category. Nor must we think of lip-reading and auditory training as two separate and distinct 'methods', the one for one type of child, the other for the other type. Each is complementary to the other and anything which will teach a child to 'communicate' is acceptable. With the child born deaf, no holds are barred.

There is still much controversy about the relative merits and demerits of each method: of lip-reading (still too often synonymous with 'oralism') and of auditory training; of 'oralism' and manualism'. But of one thing we can be quite certain. Auditory training is here to stay.

It is not surprising that 'oralism' (from the Latin word *os*, a mouth) is sometimes confused with lip-reading alone. Correctly speaking, it should refer to the general conception of 'communication by word of mouth, or by speech', and I am sure that it is used in this broader sense by most teachers of the deaf. But more and more doctors—otologists, medical officers of health, and paediatricians—are becoming interested in the problems of deafness in childhood, as they must be if we are to progress any further in early diagnosis, in prevention and possibly—is this too great a hope?—in treatment. But many doctors refer to the otologist as an 'aural' surgeon and the word 'oralism' is often confused with 'auralism'—an ugly word. The Scot, no doubt, will be able to produce two different and distinguishable vowels sounds for these two words, but the mere Sassenach (like the author) must spell them or write them if he is to draw attention to their essential differences. The spoken word 'oralism' can easily be confused, by medical audiences, with the spoken word 'auralism'; and it is to be hoped that the word 'auralism' will be banished from all future discussions on the deaf child.

Oralism versus manualism. Oralism has come for good. Very few children are born totally deaf and, given an early start, most of them can be taught 'the act of speaking to another'. This may not be enough for all their needs—educational, spiritual and emotional—but it can go a long way towards the ultimate integration of *most* deaf children into the society of their normal hearing brothers and sisters.

But we must not bury our heads in the sand. Of course there *are* failures of oralism. Of course it should not be the only method available to the really deaf child. Indeed, no less an authority than Dr Pierre Gorman has suggested that a carefully evolved system of manual gestures (in which each sign would represent a word and all the words in a phrase or sentence would be 'signed' word for word in the same sequence) might be used with advantage, in conjunction with speech and lip-reading, for communication with very young deaf children; and he believes that this would result both in a greater readiness for them to communicate in a correct linguistic form, and also in greater encouragement for them to use speech as a more meaningful mode of communication—with greater fluency of expression and with better chances of integrating themselves ultimately into the general community. 'These children,' he says, 'are being forced to use slower and more difficult forms of communication, i.e. speech and lip-reading . . . they are being made both to lose their motivation to communicate at all, and perhaps also to lose the usual forms of linguistic skills seen in the hearing group.'

'There is no evidence', says John Denmark, 'to support the contention that exposure to manual communication methods have an adverse effect upon speech and lip-reading skills'; and in 1966 G.W.G. Montgomery, Research Psychologist to Donaldson's School in Edinburgh, showed statistically that manual methods had no adverse efiects upon the development of oral skills. Furthermore, S.P. Quigley, three years later, compared two groups of deaf children, one of which had been taught by oral methods, the other by combined oral and manual methods; at the end of four years he found that there were differences in favour of the group using combined oral and manual methods, in respect of language development, speech reading and general academic achievement, and that the admission of methods of manual communication had no adverse effect on speech.

Fortunately things are changing—early diagnosis is becoming commoner; electronic equipment is more powerful and more refined; and educational techniques are improving. And as further improvements come, so it is to be hoped that the failures will be fewer, the successes more and more; and indeed many of the failures of oralism are failures of teaching, although such failures may be due, not necessarily to the method employed, but rather to failure to assess correctly all the child's difficulties.

It would be a tragedy if the relatively few failures were to detract from the main body of successes, for this could only lead to a lowering of standards. No doubt there will long remain some very deaf children for whom a combined method may offer the best chances of a full life, and there is probably much to commend it for a selected group of these children. The main difficulties are to determine who these children shall be and when manual help should be introduced; and at least we must find out, first of all, *why* some children never succeed 'orally'. But, for the majority of deaf children who are fortunate enough to have useful and usable hearing, we must aim always for the highest. And this, surely, is oralism.

Speech correction. However a deaf child may be taught to speak, his speech will always tend to show certain defects and these require constant correction. Dr Adrian Fourcin, of University College in

London, has developed a 'laryngograph', which, by monitoring the movements of the vocal cords, can help to overcome the problems of voice production and integration to profoundly deaf children.

Pre-school training. The last decade or so has witnessed great advances in the educational treatment of deafness in children: earlier diagnosis; developments in electronics; a wider recognition of the value of auditory training; and the training of more fully-qualified teachers of the deaf. All of these have brought untold benefits to many thousands of deaf children, but the most important by far has been the growing awareness of the supreme importance of correct early assessment and, through it, of early training.

It is never too early to start.

The Education Act of 1944 made provision for nursery classes in schools for the deaf for any deaf child over 2 whose parents want him to go to such a class, and there are some who think of the 'pre-school' deaf child as one under 2 years of age. Personally I prefer to think of the pre-school deaf child as one who is under the *compulsory* age of 5.

This pre-school period, this optimum period for the ecquisition of speech and language, is the most vital part of the deaf child's life, for it is in this period that the foundations of success or failure are laid. All are agreed that training should begin as soon as the handicap is recognized, and all are agreed that this should be at some time during the first two years of life, preferably in the first year.

Initially all normal children learn the basic skills of communication within their own homes. If it be accepted that deaf children also are capable of learning to communicate orally, then they too should start this in the home.

A common language is essential to communication; and this can be learned only by constant experience of speech, and by the opportunity to associate this experience with meaning. It is in the first five years of a child's life that he is most receptive to the development, not only of his relationships with others, but also of his mode of communication.

There is a need for constant repetition of speech sounds to all babies and small children, whether hearing or deaf; and this affords them adequate experience of speech itself, and the chance to associate speech with meaning.

Initially, the hearing child learns from the adults around him; but by the time he has learned to make satisfactory relationships with other children (at an average age of about $2\frac{1}{2}$), he learns better from contact with other children than with adults. The same applies to the deaf child.

Parents of the deaf child must be shown how, through the every-day routine of his home environment, he can be given the constant experience of speech that is essential if he is to learn to identify its meaning.

Pre-school training is essentially parent-training except in those very exceptional instances where the full-time services of a trained teacher of the deaf are available on an individual basis. In all other cases the mother must attend an audiology clinic where the principles of training are explained to her and where she can watch a practical demonstration of the appropriate methods, about once a week or once a fortnight. No one pretends that a teacher of the deaf can train a deaf child by these brief periods of half to three-quarters of an hour at long intervals, but she can teach the mother and answer her questions. And the mother, in her turn, can do much to train her child when circumstances are favourable. Both parents need help and guidance, and this should be provided by all of those who work in the team of an Audiology Unit or Clinic—the otologist, the teacher of the deaf and the psychologist must all be prepared to answer the many questions that occur to the bewildered parents of a deaf child. This early guidance can never be wasted and it should be continued throughout the whole of the child's school years.

It is clearly senseless to expect a mother to be able to train her deaf child if she goes out to work all day, if she is physically or mentally ill, if she has eight other children—half of them at home and half at school—or if she herself has been born deaf and does not speak. A mother can only train her deaf child if she has the intelligence and the skill and the patience and, above all, the will to train him. She must be prepared to face setbacks and she must have the temperament to accept them and overcome them. Not all mothers are made like this, and failures of home training inevitably occur.

It is never an easy matter to determine which particular children will need the full-time help that can only be provided in a special school. It is even more difficult to decide *when* a particular child is in need of this help and only regular and vigilant 'follow-up' can supply the answer, for there are so many factors—some of them immeasurable—that must be considered in deciding the issue. There are those who say that *every* deaf child should be admitted to a special school as soon as he reaches the age of 2. At the other extreme there are those who say that *no* deaf child should ever attend a special school, lest he be segregated with others who are similarly afflicted. To anyone who has had the opportunity, as I have, of seeing some of the outstanding successes (and some of the outstanding failures) of either method—of home training and of special schooling—the one view is as patently absurd as the other. Not every home is entirely satisfactory. Nor, unfortunately, is every special school. And these two factors—the home and the school—are perhaps the most difficult of many difficult and unknown 'immeasurables'. In either instance, only trial—and sometimes error—will tell.

Every child is an individual and every decision must be based on a judicious weighing of all the circumstances that operate in each and every case, and ultimately on the experience and beliefs of each and every one of those whose unenviable task it is to decide.

Schools. It is no less difficult a task to decide on the appropriate type of schooling for deaf and partially deaf (or partially hearing) children throughout the years of their school lives, from 5 to 16. But it is of the utmost importance that there be a flexible system which allows of transfers from one type to another, of upgrading or down-grading, as circumstances dictate. There is at present far too much rigidity in the system of 'placement' whereby far too often a child is 'pigeon-holed' into a set compartment. And there—come what may, succeed or fail—he stays.

There are schools for the deaf and schools for the partially hearing; there are, in certain areas, Partially Hearing Units (PHUs) attached to ordinary schools—small classes of ten children or less in the charge of a teacher of the deaf; and there are ordinary schools. There are special day schools and special residential schools; these may be primary or secondary schools, the latter including one special technical school and one special grammar school. And there are good schools and bad schools.

It may be tragic—indeed, it is tragic—to see the deaf child flounder-ing in a hearing school, frustrated daily more and more by his own sense of failure and inadequacy. But it is no less tragic to see the deaf child, almost bursting to get on, being continually held down and held back in a special school by a misplaced desire to give him 'special training'.

At the age of 5, some decision *must* be made because it is now obligatory for the parents to send their child to school. If he has no speech and no language, he is clearly in need of full-time help. But does he need the sort of help provided by the schools for the deaf, or the sort of help provided by the schools for the partially hearing? How much hearing has he? When was his deafness first detected? When was training begun—and by whom was it given? Is there a special school in his area, or will he have to leave his home? Is he a bright child or isn't he? Has he any other handicap? These and many other questions must all be answered before a decision can be made.

If he has some speech and language, he may be able to go to an ordinary school. But how much has he? And if his own speech is not yet very good, how much does he understand? It will almost certainly be more than he himself can say, but will he be able to cope with a large class of forty children? Does he live in a town where he can have extra help from time to time, from a clinic or—in a scattered population—from the peripatetic teacher? Is there a special class that he could go to in an ordinary school? Again, we must know the answers to all these questions, and many more, before we can decide.

There are many children who are obviously ready for ordinary schools; there are others who are clearly in need of special schools. But in between there are many borderline cases and it is here that the greatest difficulties arise. Whatever we decide for these children we must be prepared to review their progress—or their failure to progress—as often as time and reason permit. We must never say that this child is a 'deaf school' child and this one an 'ordinary school' child—and simply leave him there. There is a vital need for continuing re-assessment and we must be ready to move him up or move him down, much as we would within the framework of the school itself. recognizing at the same time that too many moves may be harmful. Suffice it to add that there has been a considerable growth in the number of PHUs in normal schools, and also of peripatetic teachers in both town and country areas, during the last five or six years.

The deaf child with additional handicaps

Several syndromes have recently come to light in which deafness is associated with such characteristic features as the pigmentary changes of the Waardenburg syndrome, or with other pathological states such as goitre (page 130). In none of these interesting conditions can the other features be regarded as handicaps, and in each instance the cause is some genetic weakness. But other definite handicaps can and do occur in association with inherited congential deafness and the first case of the Waardenburg syndrome I ever saw (or was aware of seeing) was associated with a congenital tracheo-oesophageal fistula (an opening between the gullet and the wind-pipe) which, despite an operation in the earliest days of her life, led to repeated bouts of pneumonia and ultimately to the little girl's death. In the absence of any known environmental cause, the association of deafness with other congenital defects (such as blindness—in the rare condition of 'retinitis pigmentosa'—or cleft palate) should always suggest a genetic cause, as also does the presence of deafness in more than one member of a family in a single generation—even in the absence of any traceable deafness in earlier generations. These so-called 'recessive' cases can also follow the inter-marriage of cousins or other related partners.

Apart from these hereditary defects, there are all too frequently other handicaps associated with the deafness due to pre-natal or perinatal influences. Two examples are maternal rubella and kernicterus.

The deafness of maternal rubella may be associated with blindness, or partial sightedness, mental deficiency or heart disease; that of kernicterus with cerebral palsy. Accordingly, deafness or partial deafness may occur with any or all of these additional handicaps, when the problems of education are enormously increased. Most deaf children depend to some extent, many to a very large extent, on visual clues but the deaf child who is also blind or partially sighted is denied this vital link with the hearing world. The 'rubella child' often presents a typical picture—staring intently through thick lenses at any light she can find, often so much more aware of light than of sound; often a fussy feeder in her earliest days, small and feeble, and sometimes very difficult to manage (Figure 16.10).

And what of the deaf child with cerebral palsy? Very often this dual handicap is caused by kernicterus, and more often than not her

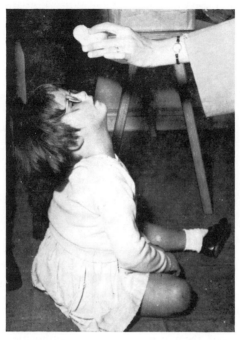

Fig. 16.10   A typical 'rubella' child.
This little girl's mother had German measles in the early months of her pregnancy. She is partially hearing and partially sighted.

executive speech difficulties are much greater than the receptive handicap of what is (characteristically) a partial high-tone deafness. The 'kernicterus child' is easily recognized by her facial grimaces, her uncertain balance, and her writhing 'athetoid' movements (Figure 16.11). Fortunately, with improvements in prevention, fewer of these unfortunate children are being seen today.

Finally, the deaf child who is also backward. Many deaf and partially-deaf children are 'educationally sub-normal', if by this term we are comparing them simply with normal children. But there are also deaf and partially-hearing children who, in addition to their hearing defect, have a defective intellectual capacity, and it is to these children that the term ESN should more commonly (and correctly) be applied.

By far the greatest difficulty facing these children with multiple handicaps—and their parents—is that of providing a satisfactory education for them. There is one special unit for the deaf and blind,

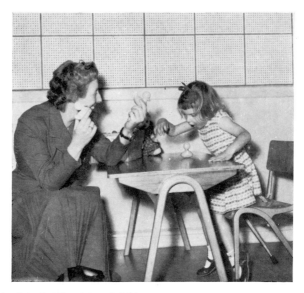

Fig. 16.11   A typical 'kernicterus' child.
The mother of this girl has Rhesus-negative blood. The child is partially deaf and
has an athetoid type of cerebral palsy. The 'balancing act' and the facial grimaces are
characteristic of this condition.

at Condover Hall in Shrewsbury; there is the GLC's School for
Partially Hearing Children with additional handicaps at Penn, in
Buckinghamshire; there are several schools for physically handicapped
children, some of them run by the local authorities, some by the
National Spastics Society; and there is now, in the London area,
a special class for partially hearing-partially sighted rubella children.
In some of them facilities exist for the full-time or part-time services
of a teacher of the deaf, who can give extra help to those children
who need it: when the physical handicap is slight, the special schools
or units for the deaf or partially hearing can usually cope with the
problem; in the case of deaf and partially-hearing ESN children, some
are accepted by the schools for the deaf and partially hearing when
they are not too backward, others by the ESN schools when the
deafness is not too great. But there is nowhere near enough provision
made for the multiply-handicapped child.

There are now in this country many special schools, each designed
to admit children suffering from one particular handicap but there
are very few which admit children with multiple handicaps. Is this a
desirable state of affairs? This question was discussed in an article on
'Special School Specialization' in *The Times Educational Supplement*
of February 21st, 1958. 'By the nature of their pupils,' writes the
correspondent, 'schools of this type collect defects additional to those
which they are established to remedy. The schools may have no one

competent to treat such secondary handicaps and, as a result, many of the children can have real needs which remain unanswered.'

This, surely, is the crux of the matter. Many teachers in the special schools are trained to deal with one handicap only. When confronted with another, they are at a loss. So also are the children. 'The bringing together of similarly affected children to the exclusion of all others can easily create a climate of living which, at best, is unstimulating'.

'It is natural but regrettable,' continues the article, 'that some staffs of special schools get anxious and may even feel wronged when children with different defects from those with which they are mainly concerned arrive at the school. It is extremely difficult for children with dual or multiple handicaps to get special school educational treatment. Staffs encounter problems in educational treatment for which they are professionally unprepared.' Would it not be better if every teacher who is training to deal, as a specialist, with one particular handicap, were to learn something first about all handicaps? And might it not be better to have special schools for handicapped children and not one for each particular type of handicapped child? The staff of such schools would include specialist teachers with different responsibilities, and secondary defects would be more likely to be discovered. For example, the partially-hearing child who was thought to be only ESN would be recognized by a teacher of the deaf far more quickly than by a teacher without such experience. No longer would a child be unacceptable to a school because of a dual disability, and most of the anomalies of placing handicapped children under the present scheme would be resolved.

'Pigeon-hole selection,' concludes the correspondent, 'is an awkward procedure which never fits the needs of human beings.'

The prevention of congenital deafness

Since there is still (regrettably) no effective remedy, either medical or surgical, for congenital perceptive deafness, the doctor must continue to focus his attention for the time being on the problems of prevention. Prevention, of course, depends upon a knowledge of causation, and it is only by continued research into the causes of congenital deafness that we shall be able (it is hoped) to take steps to prevent it. There is much still to be learnt about the causes of congenital deafness and results come slowly in this sort of work. But a great deal has been added to our knowledge in the years that have followed the Second World War, and research of this kind is being carried on continually, day in and day out, in almost every country in the world.

Medical research is always time-consuming and often heart-breaking, and no new discovery is certain of immediate rewards, for many practical difficulties may stand in our way before new knowledge can be translated into terms of practical Preventive Medicine. We know, for example, that congenital deafness can be caused by genetic weakness. We have known this for a very long time, yet the only available method of preventing this type of deafness (by purely medical or surgical means) is by sterilization—objectionable to some on moral grounds. Have we not, only too recently, witnessed the attempts of one man to breed a 'pure' race? Nor would we recommend such a method when we do not even know the extent of the risk. To quote from an article in *Medical World*, published in August 1958: 'If a child has inherited deafness from one or both of his parents, or from one of his more distant relatives, there is always a distinct risk that he will pass on the 'bad seed' to his own offspring. The chances of handing down this genetic weakness to subsequent generations can never be forecast with mathematical precision, but we can be quite certain that if such a child grows up and marries another who has inherited the same genetic weakness from *her* ancestors, the risk will be enormously increased. This applies, though to a lesser extent, to the intermarriage of cousins, for recessive genes are much more likely to be transmitted by blood relations. All such unions should therefore be discouraged.' In these cases of hereditary congenital deafness, the doctor's main role is one of 'marriage counsellor'.

There can be no doubt that if more deaf adults were more fully integrated into hearing society, there would be less inter-marriage among the deaf, and if the 'bad seed' could thus be weakened fewer children would be born deaf. But this ideal is far removed from present reality, and most of our efforts must be concentrated on preventing those other forms of congenital deafness which arise from environmental influences—mainly from rubella and kernicterus.

German measles is a mild infection and a single attack will often, but not by any means always, confer a lasting immunity. If we could guarantee that every female child would contract rubella before she reached the age of child-bearing, we could be almost certain that congenital deafness from this cause would be wiped away. There have been many campaigns to expose girls to the infection during their school years but unfortunately this does not always work. When my own two daughters had German measles we 'imported' two of their cousins from Hampshire. They slept not only in the same room but even in the same beds, yet still they returned to the edge of the New Forest unmarked and unprotected. There must therefore remain a number of women who will come into contact with rubella unprotected, during the early months of pregnancy.

In 1954 a 'gamma-globulin' was made available to all doctors in Britain, and it was suggested that it should be given without delay to every pregnant woman who had had the rash or been in contact with it. Although these injections have been shown to afford at least some degree of protection to the recipient, it has not yet been established whether or not they protect the fetus. However this may be, it is now known that gamma-globulins are uncertain in their effects; and this would point to the need for a vaccine. Such a vaccine is now available for school girls from the age of thirteen years onwards, but this is not yet statutory, consent resting with the parents.

It must be remembered that congenital defects may sometimes follow a 'sub-clinical' attack of rubella, and I have seen one typical 'rubella' child with congenital deafness whose mother had had only the very vaguest of indirect contacts with the virus. After long and careful reflection her husband (a taxi-driver in Oxford) had remembered that, at some time during the early part of her pregnancy, he had been commissioned to take a group of spotty schoolgirls from their school to their homes. Neither he nor his wife had had a rash.

On purely medical grounds there is clearly something to be said for terminating a pregnancy which has been complicated by rubella, but there are many other factors to be considered, both legal and moral.

The discovery of the Rhesus blood groups has helped to prevent many cases of congenital deafness—and cerebral palsy—and the incidence of deafness from this cause has now been greatly reduced. Since the deafness in these cases is due to the jaundice, and the jaundice is rarely evident until hours or days after birth, every effort must be made to replace the child's blood completely and immediately, before any sign of jaundice appears.

17. Acquired Sensori-neural Deafness

Traumatic sensori-neural deafness

The term 'trauma' is used, in the present context, to embrace head injuries, pressure changes affecting the inner ear, and exposure to excessive noise.

Perceptive deafness may follow injuries to the head, and not uncommonly it is associated with fractures involving the base of the skull.

Sensori-neural deafness due to head injuries

Fractures of the skull base

These fractures more commonly involve the middle ear, to produce a conductive deafness (page 84) but occasionally the line of fracture passes through the inner ear or the internal auditory canal, to produce haemorrhage into the cochlea or vestibular labyrinth, or the internal canal. The organ of Corti may be ruptured, or the bony spiral lamina fractured. The fracture may be so minute that it is invisible on X-rays, but more extensive fractures can usually be demonstrated radiographically. Basal fractures which are extensive enough to involve both ears are rarely compatible with survival, and these cases normally present clinically with unilateral sensori-neural deafness. There may, however, be some loss of hearing on the side opposite to the one mainly affected. The deafness in the worse ear is usually severe and permanent.

Concussion of the labyrinth

This may also follow falls or blows on the skull or jaws and is distinguished from fractures of the skull by the temporary nature of the hearing loss. It results from the same type of injury, but no fracture is seen on X-ray and the hearing loss is less severe, commonly causing a V-shaped 'dip' at 4000 Hz on the pure tone audiogram. It usually recovers in a few days but may persist for weeks or months, and if the deafness remains unchanged for six months or more, it must be assumed that a microscopical fracture has occurred and that the deafness is therefore likely to be permanent.

Sensori-neural deafness due to pressure changes

Blast injuries of the inner ear

A blast wave has two phases—a primary wave of increased pressure, followed by a secondary wave of decreased pressure. The secondary wave is weaker than the primary wave, but it lasts longer; and it is this secondary wave which damages the inner ear, by producing a haemorrhage into the labyrinth or a rupture of the organ of Corti.

Blast and explosions may damage the middle ear or the inner ear, or both, but a pure conductive deafness is rare. It is the extent of damage to the inner ear which determines the final degree of disability following these injuries, and it used to be thought that a rupture of the tympanic membrane exerted some protective influence on the inner ear. In other words, that the sensori-neural deafness tended to be worse when the membrane remained intact, less severe when it was ruptured. However, this view has recently been challenged. There is usually some recovery in hearing after blast injuries to the ear but any deafness that does persist for more than six months is likely to be perceptive—and permanent. On the other hand there may also be a slow, progressive degeneration of the hair-cells even after apparent recovery and this may easily be confused with a premature 'senile' deafness.

Tinnitus and vertigo are common but usually disappear.

Barotraumatic otitis interna

'Barotrauma' most commonly affects the middle ear cleft (see page 87) but rarely a sensori-neural deafness may be caused by subjection to a raised atmospheric pressure, and it may be severe and permanent.

Round window rupture

Victor Goodhill, of Los Angeles, has drawn our attention to spontaneous rupture of the round window membrane following a rise of intracranial pressure, for example by coughing, sneezing, straining or physical exertion; and it is possible that sudden changes in middle ear pressure, as after air travel, may result in a similar lesion.

Sensori-neural deafness due to noise

In 1831 Fosbroke described deafness occurring in blacksmiths, and in 1890 Barr surveyed 100 boilermakers who had worked at their trade for more than three or four years. Not one of them had normal hearing, and for more than half a century 'boilermaker's deafness' remained the classical example of noise-induced hearing loss. Many other occupations have been added in the intervening years, and the mid-twentieth century has witnessed another addition in the form of the jet engine.

Noise-induced deafness is of two types—the acute and the chronic.

The acute type can be caused by a wide variety of 'acoustic shocks' (or impulse noises), such as the nearby detonation of fireworks or small-arms fire, atmospheric and other disturbances in the receivers of telephones, or the high-pitched shriek of a whistle. The deafness of rifle shooting is more marked in the left ear in the right-shouldered shot, since the butt of the rifle is nearer to this ear, and the audiogram (Figure 17.1) shows the typical V-shaped 'dip' at 4000 Hz so commonly associated with many forms of traumatic sensori-neural deafness. This type is known as *acoustic trauma*.

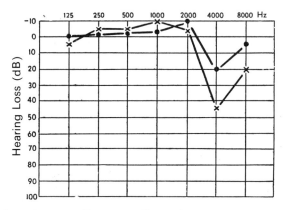

Fig. 17.1 Acoustic trauma. (Pure tone audiogram.)
The patient is one of Britain's leading authorities on poliomyelitis, and for many years he has been a keen small-arms shot. The audiogram shows a typical 'dip' at 4000 Hz, more marked (in a right-shouldered shot) in the left ear.

The chronic type of noise trauma follows prolonged exposure to high intensity-levels of noise and is usually referred to as *industrial noise-induced hearing loss*. It occurs in boilermakers, drop-forge workers, shippers and riveters, stampers, platers, headers, welders, wormers, turners, and those who work with pneumatic drills; it is also found in petrol or jet aircraft workers, whether in the cabin or on the ground. According to Lieut.-Colonel J. E. Lett, of the United States Army Air Force School of Aviation Medicine, the noise of a jet engine is now the loudest industrial noise, measuring between 120 and 140 dB above threshold level. The effects of noise are always worse in enclosed spaces, and the degree of deafness varies with its intensity and the duration of exposure. A level above 90 dB (or even 85 dB) is considered to be 'unsafe' and high-frequency noise is more harmful than low-frequency noise. There is also a marked individual susceptibility to noise and it is of the utmost importance that all personnel should be 'screened' before employment in noisy industries.

More recently there have been reports of high-frequency sensori-neural deafness caused by exposure (of dentists) to high-speed dental drills, and it has also been shown that some 'pop' musicians may suffer from noise-induced hearing loss; but this has not been reported in classical orchestral players. Although it is vehemently denied by some authorities, others are still concerned about the possibility of damage from the enormous power output of certain modern hearing aids, some of them reaching a level as high as 148 dB.

With the exception of head injuries with fractures of the skull base (when the hearing loss tends to be severe and permanent), the characteristic feature of most cases of traumatic sensorineural deafness is a high-tone hearing loss, often with a marked V-shaped 'dip' and greatest at a frequency of about 4000 Hz. It is thought by some that this 'dip' at 4000 Hz is due to the fact that the part of the cochlea which receives and analyses these higher tones is situated near to the labyrinthine windows, at the base of the cochlea, and that it is this proximity of the basal turns of the cochlea to the windows which makes them more exposed (and therefore more vulnerable) to sound waves of high intensity.

The problem of industrial noise is a growing one, but much work is being done to minimize its worst effects.

Noise and the law

In a written answer in the House of Commons on 31 October 1973 Sir Keith Joseph, then Secretary of State for Social Services, said that he accepted the recommendations made in the report of the Industrial Injuries Advisory Panel on occupational deafness. Their report was published in November 1973 and it recommended that noise-induced deafness should be 'prescribed' as an industrial disease within the meaning of the National Insurance (Industrial Injuries) Act of 1965 but that initially it should be limited to at least twenty years' exposure to those industrial processes which produced the highest levels of noise; these are drop-forging and the use of pneumatic tools in the metal-manufacturing and the ship-building and repairing industries.

This recommendation was implemented in October 1974, when occupational deafness was added to the list of prescribed industrial diseases, with effect from 5 February 1975.

To qualify for compensation, a claimant must show that he has worked for twenty years or more in any occupation involving 'the use of pneumatic percussive tools or high speed grinding tools in the cleaning, dressing or finishing of ingots, billets or blooms'; or 'the use of pneumatic tools on metal in the ship-building and ship-repairing industries'; or 'work wholly or mainly in the immediate vicinity of drop-forging plant or forging press plant engaged in the shaping of hot metals'.

For the purposes of such benefit, occupational deafness is defined as 'substantial permanent sensori-neural hearing loss due to occupational noise amounting to at least 50 dB in the *better* ear, being the average . . . of pure tone losses measured by audiometry over the 1, 2 and 3 kHz frequencies', after the exclusion of hearing losses due to any factors other than occupational noise.

This minimum hearing loss is rated at 20 per cent disablement, more severe losses being rated proportionately higher; and claims must be made not later than one year after the cessation of such employment.

These terms are by no means over generous, but they do represent a new and major step forward concerning industrial injuries, and it has been recommended that this initial scheme should be extended gradually to other noisy industries and occupations.

Sensori-neural deafness due to infections

Severe sensori-neural deafness may result from almost any of the common infectious fevers, particularly in childhood, and of these measles, mumps and meningitis are most often responsible.

Apart from a conductive deafness due to otitis media, measles may also cause a sensori-neural deafness due to the toxic effects of the virus, and in such cases there is usually a partial deafness of moderately severe degree in both ears, with a tendency to affect the high tones slightly more than the low tones. There is therefore a gently-sloping audiogram at an average level of about 45–50 dB (Figure 17.2).

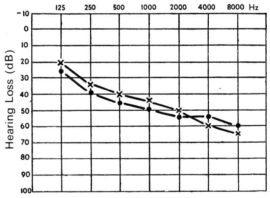

Fig. 17.2   Acquired sensori-neural deafness due to measles. (Pure tone audiogram). The curve slopes gently downwards to the right.

The characteristic deafness of mumps is a unilateral sensori-neural loss which leaves the affected ear totally deaf and the other perfectly normal. The audiogram in Figure 6.5 (p. 44) shows the typical response of a severe unilateral sensori-neural deafness (see page 43).

Some of the severest cases of deafness ever seen are those which result from meningitis, and not uncommonly it is total or almost total (Figure 17.3). Many of these cases complicate the tuberculous

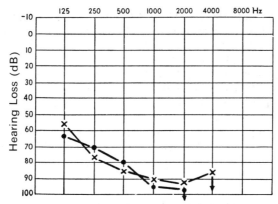

Fig. 17.3   Acquired sensori-neural deafness due to meningitis. (Pure tone audiogram.) Post-meningitic deafness tends to be extremely severe.

type of meningeal infection but deafness may also follow other types of meningitis. There is still some controversy as to whether the deafness results from the meningitis itself, or from the streptomycin which was used, almost universally in the treatment of tuberculous meningeal infections (see page 189) until alternative anti-tuberculous drugs were discovered.

There is much to commend the routine application of hearing tests, including audiometry where possible, in all patients who have suffered from these three particular infectious illnesses.

Scarlet fever and influenza are much less common causes, and typhoid is very rare in this country. Syphilis is not so rare as is often supposed and it is a cause that must never be forgotten, especially as this 'great mimic' can produce almost any 'pattern' of sensori-neural (or conductive) deafness.

Characteristically the natural history of syphilitic deafness is one of slow relentless progression to profound bilateral deafness, with occasional fluctuations and not infrequently sudden loss.

Once in a while one sees a small crop of cases of sensori-neural deafness due to 'otitic herpes', in which the deafness may form part of a more widespread symptom-complex (the Ramsay-Hunt syndrome). It is a form of herpes zoster (or 'shingles'), in which earache is followed (often after many days) by a rash (of vesicles, or 'blisters') in and around the ear. Facial paralysis may appear suddenly, and the deafness is probably due to spread of the infection to the spiral ganglion (page 11). It is a virus infection which occurs in epidemics, most commonly in the summer or autumn, and there is reason to believe that the virus is identical with that of chicken-pox. It is also communicable and not uncommonly occurs in those who have been in contact with established cases of chicken-pox, usually after an incubation period of about two weeks.

Otitic labyrinthitis is usually caused by direct spread of infection from the middle ear to the inner ear, usually during an acute exacerbation of a long-standing chronic infection of the middle ear cleft, and almost always in association with cholesteatoma. Occasionally the infection enters the inner ear through the oval or round window, much more commonly through erosion of the bony horizontal semicircular canal. In the worst cases, the inner ear is overthrown by a severe suppurative infection which causes violent vertigo and permanent sensori-neural deafness. Less often, suppurative labyrinthitis may result from cerebro-spinal fever, or from infection secondary to fractures of the skull base.

Much more doubtful is the role of the 'septic focus'. It was at one time thought that sensori-neural deafness could be reversed sometimes by removal of a focus of chronic infection in the tonsils, teeth, nasal sinuses, or gall-bladder. But this is extremely doubtful, and in any event there are few otologists today who would remove or drain these structures unless there were some very definite local indication for such intervention.

Cochlear otosclerosis

Pure cochlear otosclerosis is characterized by a progressive sensorineural hearing loss, usually bilateral and usually symmetrical. The progression is usually slow, and the hearing tends to remain stationary for quite long periods of time. The age of onset of the deafness is similar to that of the much commoner stapedial variety. The high tones are usually affected more than the low tones, and the disease may be demonstrable radiographically.

Cogan's disease

This rare disease, which was first described by Cogan in 1949, is characterized by a fluctuating and progressive sensori-neural hearing loss associated with non-syphilitic interstitial keratitis of the eyes and not uncommonly with vestibular disturbances. The clinical features of Cogan's disease are almost indistinguishable from those of late syphilis, and the pathological changes in the temporal bones are very similar. It may have an 'auto-immune' basis, and it is thought that the deafness, which may progress to a total bilateral hearing loss, may sometimes be arrested by early treatment with steroids. This, of course, demands early diagnosis and the condition is one that should be suspected, despite its great rarity, in any unexplained case of progressive bilateral sensori-neural hearing loss.

Deafness due to drugs

'The phenomenon of ototoxic deafness must be at least as old as the use of wormseed and Peruvian bark in the pre-Columbian pharmacopoeia of the Americas. Unfortunately, the documentation from that high and far-off time is scanty at best, and the names of the Shamans who first remarked on the evil influence of chenopodium oil and the cinchona alkaloids on their patients' hearing are lost in the dawn mists of pre-history . . . Although salicylate ototoxicity is presumably more recent, it too is of a respectable antiquity . . . It has remained for this generation to develop . . . therapeutic agents of highly specific, permanent ototoxic effect. These are the basic antibiotics'.

Thus wrote Dr Joseph Hawkins in 1967, and it summarizes very well the history of deafness due to drugs.

Quinine and other 'cinchona alkaloids' were indeed used by the medicine men (Shamans) of the North American Indians long before the occupation by white settlers of that vast continent which is celebrating the bicentenary of its independence at the time of writing; and the salicylates (including Aspirin and its many derivatives and compounds) continue to be amongst the most effective and widely-used drugs available.

It is almost certain that 'ototoxicity' has been present since drugs were first used and, although it is better known for its stunting effect on the growth of limbs, it was thalidomide (which can also cause deafness, either conductive or—less commonly—sensori-neural) that first drew widespread public attention to the potentially harmful effects of drugs.

But in relation to toxic deafness, it is the diuretics (such as frusemide and ethacrynic acid) and particularly the 'unruly family of basic streptomyces antibiotics' (Hawkins) which cause us the greatest concern. These amino-glycoside antibiotics include streptomycin, neomycin, kanamycin and gentamicin—all of them still widely used in clinical practice. Although their adverse effects are much more serious and much more predictable when they are administered systemically—that is, by injection or even by mouth—they may also produce their toxic effects when they are applied topically, not least to the ears themselves, usually in the form of drops.

It would be irresponsible to exaggerate the ototoxicity of these life-saving drugs, but they should never be used lightly or without careful thought, because they *can* produce deafness—always sensori-neural, often severe, and always irreversible—and their use should be limited to the treatment of those infections which do not respond to other less toxic preparations.

The deafness is usually preceded by tinnitus, which should always be regarded as a warning sign of impending hearing loss; and it may develop as long as several months after the completion of treatment. It is more likely to occur in the very young and the very old; it is more likely to occur in the presence of kidney or liver disease; and it can affect an unborn child when these drugs are given to a pregnant mother.

It is vitally important, therefore, that no drugs which are known to be potentially toxic to the ears and hearing should be prescribed unless there is no satisfactory alternative.

Acoustic tumours

It is a strange but interesting fact that no primary tumour, either benign or malignant, has ever been known to arise in the inner ear itself. There are, however, many records of the rather rare 'benign' tumour which arises from the sheath of the auditory nerve—benign only in so far as it does not spread to distant sites; highly dangerous in that it grows locally to invade the surrounding structures in this most important region, with paralysis of function of neighbouring cranial nerves and a high operative mortality-rate in late cases. Early diagnosis is therefore of the utmost importance and it is of particular significance to the otologist that the first symptoms are otological.

Tinnitus or sensorineural deafness is the first symptom in many cases of VIIIth nerve tumour, but it is nearly always unilateral and is often so severe when it is first seen by the otologist (or noticed by the patient) that it may be confused with a simple conductive deafness (page 40). The occasional occurrence of a true conductive deafness in its early stages has added to this confusion.

Although it may progress suddenly in rare instances, the deafness is usually insidious in onset and progresses very slowly. It may remain the only symptom (indeed it may not even be noticed) for a long time, and it is probably the slow rate of progression in most cases that causes the patient so often to wait for the onset of other neurological symptoms before he seeks advice. These include unsteadiness of gait or involvement of other cranial nerves, but by this time the tumour is usually large and the outlook accordingly poorer.

Even in the very best of hands there is a significant immediate post-operative mortality in late cases, but the tumour can be removed *in toto*, if the surgeon is given the opportunity to operate when the symptoms are still entirely otological, especially by newer approaches through the inner ear or the middle fossa of the skull. It is therefore the onerous responsibility of the otologist to recognize these tumours early, in those all-too-few instances where his advice is sought when deafness alone is present.

Recruitment of loudness (page 36) is thought to be characteristic of a sensorineural deafness due to some lesion of the end-organ, but it may also occur, rarely, in acoustic tumours. Its absence, however, is almost confirmatory of a 'central' type of deafness, which will include many of these tumours. Radiographic examination may show expansion of the internal auditory canal (Figure 17.4), and other investigations (of vestibular function and of the protein content of the cerebrospinal fluid) will often produce valuable corroborative evidence. But it is deafness (or tinnitus) which is most commonly

R   L

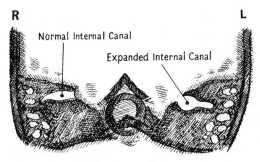

Fig. 17.4   Acoustic tumour—drawing from an X-ray.
A tumour of the left auditory nerve has expanded the internal auditory canal, through which the nerve passes from the inner ear to the brain stem.

the presenting symptom, and it is at this very early stage that the condition should be diagnosed if the patient is to be given the best chance of survival without serious, and often disfiguring, complications.

Menière's disease

Prosper Menière was a French physician who lived from 1799 to 1862, and it was in the year before his death that he wrote, in the *Gazette Médicale de Paris,* that: 'I have spoken elsewhere, a long time ago, of a girl who journeying on the box-seat of a stage coach, became as a result of the severe cold suddenly and completely deaf'. Her principal symptom was a continuous vertigo, greatly aggravated by movement. She died on the fifth day. At the post-mortem examination, the only lesion was 'a red, plastic matter, a sort of bloody exudate' in the semicircular canals.

For many years, this association of deafness and vertigo was thought to be due to a haemorrhage into the inner ear and, indeed, this may occur rarely in cases of leukaemia. I have also seen it in a haemophiliac subject who became totally deaf in his right ear after the left external carotid artery had been ligatured for an otherwise uncontrollable bleeding after tonsillectomy. It was not until 1938 that Dr C. S. Hallpike and the late Sir Hugh Cairns demonstrated an obstructive distension of the whole of the inner, endolymphatic tubular system of the labyrinth in a typical case of what is now called 'Menière's disease' (Figure 17.5). Hence the disease which now (by common consent) bears his name is not the same as the disease originally described by Menière himself. But 'the importance of Menière's original observation,' say Scott Stevenson and Guthrie, 'was that until then vertigo had been looked upon as denoting an intracranial disorder, and he showed that it could be due to an affection of the internal ear.'

Menière's disease, or endolymphatic hydrops, usually begins between the ages of 35 and 55, and its most distressing feature is the occurrence

Dilated Scala Media

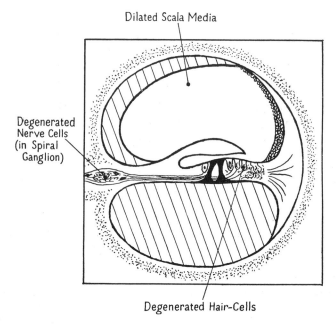

Degenerated
Nerve Cells
(in Spiral
Ganglion)

Degenerated Hair-Cells

Fig. 17.5   Menière's disease. (Microscopic section of cochlea.)
The scala media (the membranous inner tube) is grossly dilated, with marked displacement of Reissner's membrane (compare with Fig. 2.6). There is degeneration of the
hair-cells of the organ of Corti, and of the nerve cells in the spiral ganglion.

of recurring attacks of severe and crippling vertigo. These are usually
described as a sense of rotation, often accompanied by nausea and
sometimes by vomiting. But it is the deafness which concerns us here.

It is usually unilateral, although it tends ultimately to become
bilateral in about 20 per cent of cases or more. 'Some degree of
deafness in one ear,' said the late Sir Terence Cawthorne, 'is the rule
in Menière's disease.' And he points out that it precedes the vertigo
in about a half of all cases; in the other half, it is noticed either with
the first attack of vertigo, or much more rarely, after several attacks.
The hearing may improve between the attacks, and there are a few
cases in which typical attacks occur over several years with normal
hearing between attacks. Lermoyez describes this type as 'the vertigo
that makes one hear'. Usually, the hearing loss affects low tones
before the high tones, but on the whole the deafness' of Menière's
disease is a recruiting sensori-neural deafness, and it tends to progress
with each succeeding attack.

It has been said that the disease will often 'burn itself out' and that
when the deafness is total, there will be no further attacks of vertigo.
This certainly does not happen as often as is commonly supposed.

Since the deafness may often precede the vertiginous attacks, sometimes by several years, is there any feature which allows us to diagnose Menière's disease in the patient who presents himself with a unilateral (or more rarely a bilateral) sensori-neural deafness? Cawthorne emphasized that there is often an element of distortion which makes it uncomfortable for the sufferer to listen to music and makes him unduly sensitive to such sounds as the rattling of crockery, or the cries of children. He also pointed out that there is often an uncomfortable sense of fullness around the affected ear. Furthermore, the presence of a low-tone hearing-loss in a patient with sensorineural deafness is always suggestive of Menière's disease.

Senile deafness – Presbyacusis

It is always rather embarrassing to tell a man in his early fifties that he is suffering from senile deafness. But this is, for better or for worse, the term usually applied to that type of progressive sensori-neural deafness which comes on and advances, for no apparent reason, with the years.

It is due to an atrophy of the hair-cells and auditory nerve fibres in the cochlea, and is most commonly noticed around the age of 60. But a premature onset may be associated with bouts of otitis media in childhood and (particularly) with prolonged exposure to noise throughout a working life. We know very little about senile deafness, beyond the facts that it is progressive; it is sometimes, but not always, associated with high blood pressure or general atherosclerosis; and it is characteristically a *recruiting* deafness. High tones are affected first and foremost, and hearing by bone conduction is reduced, often grossly so. The singing of birds and the ringing of bells are lost first, but speech is also difficult to follow, especially when it is rapid speech. Group conversation becomes impossible, particularly in noisy surroundings, and a general slowing of the central reaction time makes matters no easier.

But there may be no other evidence of 'senility', and F. W. Watkyn-Thomas observed that 'a high degree of deafness, presumably senile, is perfectly and frequently compatible with alert and vigorous old age; on the other hand, subjects in other respects lamentably senile preserve excellent hearing'.

'Ecclesiastes,' he added, 'reminds us that our senses decay with the years. Hearing is the youngest of the special senses and, on the general principle of neurology that the last function to come is the first to go, it should be the most vulnerable. But there is more to it than this. Of all the senses, hearing is the most continuously insulted by engineers and other makers and lovers of noises. We shut our eyes against a glare or put on coloured glasses; the sense of smell is, mercifully, quickly and easily fatigued; hearing is inadequately protected by nature in a mechanized world and, outside the Fighting

Services, it is seldom protected by art. We must remember that the majority of men now in their sixth and seventh decades have been engaged in at least one war as well as other noisy activities, and a large majority have indulged excessively in tobacco. Add to these the cumulative effects of possible dental and other sepsis, and we realize that it is amazing that hearing survives as long and as well as it usually does.'

Unilateral sensori-neural deafness

The clinical features and diagnostic pitfalls of unilateral perceptive deafness have already been considered in some detail (page 43). The handicap is, of course, less severe than that of bilateral deafness but there *is* a handicap, both educationally and socially. Unilateral deafness, however severe, should have little effect on a child's educational progress provided that it is recognized and the child allowed to sit near the front of his class, with his good ear towards the teacher. But he may miss quite a lot if he is sitting near the back of the class with his bad ear towards his teacher and the hearing in the good ear is masked by the usual background noises of a big and busy classroom. In the adult, the main handicap of a severe unilateral deafness is a social one. The hearing is adequate for everyday conversation but difficulty is experienced at such social functions as dinners, where a fixed place is allotted; with the usual clatter of plates and hum of conversation (heard in the good ear), hearing may be impossible in the affected one.

But there is more to it than that, for unilateral sensori-neural deafness may be a vitally important and early symptom of certain dangerous conditions which may even prove fatal if not recognized at this stage when deafness is the only symptom (page 40). It therefore behoves the otologist to acquaint himself with the causes of this not very common type of deafness.

The cause is usually obvious when the deafness follows a head injury, especially when there is definite radiographic evidence of a fracture; nor has one to look far when a 'labyrinthine storm' occurs in a person with long-standing suppuration of the middle ear cleft. Congenital syphilis, uncommon though it is today, should still always suggest itself when an adolescent becomes suddenly deaf, in one ear or in both, sometimes overnight; and some form of vascular occlusion is often to be suspected when an adult is overcome by sudden deafness, usually in one ear. This may be associated with a raised blood pressure or with some disorder of the blood itself, especially leukaemia. The rash of an otitic herpes may be very short-lived, and the only concrete evidence of the cause may therefore be missing when the patient comes to seek advice about his hearing.

But the most perplexing cases of unilateral sensori-neural deafness are those which occur in small children, or progress insidiously. By far the commonest cause in children is mumps, and the deafness can occur at any age. Because of the general disturbances of the illness and the youth of these patients, the deafness (affecting, as it does, only one ear) will very often go unnoticed for a long time, sometimes for years; but the parents will often agree, in response to direct questioning, that they had noticed for some time that their child had tended to turn his good ear when spoken to. Doctors Jackson and Fisch drew our attention to the occurrence of unilateral deafness in children who had been born deaf through maternal rubella. In a carefully controlled group of 57 children whose mothers had had rubella during the first four months of pregnancy, no less than 30 per cent were born with some degree of deafness, usually partial. And in one out of every three of these, the deafness (always sensori-neural) was unilateral.

We must always think of the possibility of Menière's disease when an adult patient presents himself with a sensori-neural deafness in one ear, especially when the tympanic membrane is normal, when there is no history of injury, when the onset is gradual, and (in particular) when there is a hypersensitivity to noise. In such cases, the deafness may precede the attacks of vertigo by months or even years. But a similar type of progressive deafness, often affecting the high tones first, may also occur as the earliest symptom of an acoustic tumour, and no examination is complete without radiological examination of the skull and complete tests of cochlear and vestibular function.

Deafness is a common symptom of a wide variety of conditions, all of them important, some of them dangerous. This applies particularly to cases of unilateral deafness, and we must never dismiss them lightly. Whenever we are in doubt as to the cause of a unilateral deafness, whether sensori-neural or conductive, we should see the patient from time to time, to check on the progress of his hearing loss. Considerable variations can occur in Menière's disease, but we must never forget the possibility of a functional deafness, especially malingering (page 205) when the deafness follows an injury, and litigation is 'in the air'.

Sensori-neural deafness of sudden onset

The rapid onset of deafness is always alarming, whether it affects both ears or only one. The onset may be instantaneous, or the loss may progress over hours or days. A roaring tinnitus may accompany the deafness, and vertigo is not uncommon. Apart from the cases associated with wax or infections of the middle ear cleft (including those rare cases which are due to compression of the Eustachian tube in new growths of the nasopharynx), sudden deafness is nearly always due to some affection of the neural apparatus of hearing—either the cochlea itself, or the auditory nerve and its connections.

Toxic neuritis may be caused by any of several infections, including measles, mumps, scarlet fever, and herpes; and reports have appeared of so-called epidemics of unilateral sensori-neural deafness occurring in limited geographical areas and recovering spontaneously. They may have been caused by an encephalitis. Nerve deafness may appear quite suddenly in suppurative labyrinthitis or meningitis; and congenital syphilis is another cause that is all too easily forgotten. Sudden deafness may also result from an 'anaphylactic' reaction to the injection of a vaccine; and in a paper by O. E. Hallberg, in the United States, he described two patients in which a bee-sting was thought to be responsible. Transfusion with Rhesus-incompatible blood has been named as a cause by E. P. Fowler; and a further cause is spontaneous haemorrhage into the labyrinth in such blood diseases as leukaemia. A traumatic origin is usually obvious, especially where deafness follows a fracture of the skull base.

Deafness from these causes is nearly always sudden, severe and permanent. By contrast the deafness of Menière's disease tends to fluctuate and to take second place, at least in the patient's estimation, to the crippling attacks of vertigo. Hysteria is a rare cause of sudden deafness, but its possibility should always be borne in mind, especially when the deafness is bilateral; malingering should be suspected in the potential litigant, who usually feigns a unilateral deafness.

Fowler has remarked that sudden deafness of unknown origin is commoner, in his experience, than sudden deafness of known origin. 'Sudden unilateral or bilateral impairment of hearing' says Hallberg, 'is a symptom, not a disease'; and it behoves us to seek the cause, especially as treatment may succeed if the mechanism is understood and the patient seen early.

Hallberg recorded his experience of 178 patients with deafness of sudden onset who were seen at the Mayo Clinic in the five years from 1949 to 1953. In no less than 89 of these, no apparent cause was found but all of them had a sensorineural deafness, usually of the end-organ type, with recruitment of loudness; and this finding is quite compatible with the commonly held view that most of these cases have a vascular origin. The cochlear (and the vestibular) branches of the internal auditory artery are 'end-arteries'—that is to say, they make no connection with others—and thrombosis, haemorrhage or vasospasm can therefore affect the end-organ, to produce sudden deafness, total or partial. Of the 89 patients whom Hallberg classified as probably of vascular origin, about a quarter had high blood pressure, or atherosclerosis, or both. The majority were in the older age-group, and the age distribution accorded fairly closely with that of coronary occlusion. There was some evidence that such patients were abnormally susceptible to other types of vascular accident later in life.

'In such a fine mechanism as that of the end-organ of hearing,' said Hallberg, 'irreversible changes may take place quickly.' It is not surprising, therefore, that the deafness is often permanent. Andrew Morrison has emphasized that the deafness of an acoustic tumour may also be sudden in onset.

The prevention and management of acquired sensori-neural deafness

There is a limited number of cases of sensori-neural deafness in which the hearing loss may vary considerably, and a further limited number in which recovery may occur spontaneously, either in whole or in part. There is even a small number in which we may actually be able to do something about it. But it is regrettably true to say that little or nothing can be done to improve the hearing, by medical or surgical means, in the majority of cases of sensori-neural deafness.

There is often a marked fluctuation in hearing in cases of Menière's disease, and this is also a characteristic feature in cases of functional deafness. Recovery is expected in concussion of the labyrinth, and it may occur in cases of industrial noise-induced hearing loss—if the susceptible subject be removed early enough from the exciting cause. The onset of deafness is usually insidious in these workers, and it is important that we should be able to detect the susceptible individual before symptoms arise—indeed, before any man is accepted for employment in the noisier industries. Air Vice-Marshal E. D. D. Dickson believes that some idea of susceptibility could be gained if we knew at what rate the hearing recovered, in any one person, after a period of exposure; and W. E. Grove has recommended that every workman engaged in a job where the noise level exceeds 90 decibels above threshold should have a pre-employment audiogram and be re-tested after one week, and subsequently at regular intervals. Any workman who complains of tinnitus after working in a noisy environment should also have his hearing re-tested.

Colin Johnston, who investigated the hearing of over 200 workmen in the industrial Midlands, has observed that the ideal remedy would be to eliminate the injurious noise. Improvement in the design of machines and their mountings has already done much to help; and reduction of reflection and reverberation of noise by sound-proofing surfaces and baffle walls has sometimes been effective. Failing these measures, there remains the 'acoustic insulation' of the workers' ears by protective devices, and Johnston found that of 64 boilermakers only 10 wore protective devices in the ears, but in no other trade were they worn at all. An ear plug, such as cotton-wool impregnated with yellow soft paraffin, may attenuate noise by 20–30 decibels; and simple ear plugs of soft silicone rubber (Figure 17.6) may give a noise attenuation of 15–35 decibels, depending upon the frequency of the stimulating noise. However, the most effective protection is afforded by covering the ears completely with an 'ear defender' (Figure 17.7), which may attenuate noise by as much as 35–45 decibels in the most

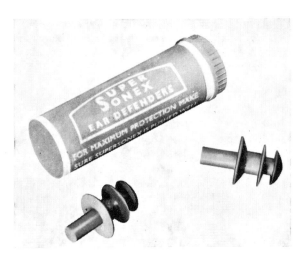

Fig. 17.6   Ear plugs. *(By courtesy of Racal-Amplivox Communications Ltd., Safety Product Division)*

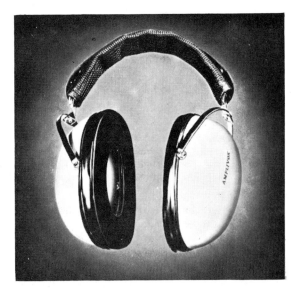

Fig. 17.7   Hearing protectors. *(By courtesy of Racal-Amplivox Communicatiohs Ltd. Safety Product Division.)*

vulnerable frequencies. These devices, of course, must also reduce the wearer's hearing for conversation, but their use should be encouraged in those Service personnel and industrial workers who are constantly exposed to very high intensities.

Those who shoot regularly should use ear plugs whenever they shoot, and the so-called 'gun-fenders' have been found to afford good protection, whilst still allowing the wearer to carry on a conversation and to hear the sounds of birds rising.

It is very doubtful whether sensori-neural deafness is ever caused by absorption of toxins from a 'septic focus' and there is rarely any indication for the removal (on this account) of infected teeth, tonsils or gall-bladder.

But deafness *can* be caused by certain drugs, and it is wise to withdraw any ototoxic drug whenever there is audiometric evidence of a hearing loss, unless there is no satisfactory alternative. The aminoglycoside antibiotics in particular should be avoided altogether unless they are essential to the patient's survival or subsequent well-being, especially in cases of kidney or liver disease, and in the very young or the very old; and they should be avoided whenever possible in pregnant women.

Several years ago it was discovered that there was a significantly higher incidence of cochlear otosclerosis in some areas of the United States than in others; and careful comparison of the water supplies in these different areas showed that it was considerably commoner in those areas in which the fluoride content of the drinking water was low. Fluorides have since been used in the treatment of this otherwise untreatable form of otosclerosis, with some reported successes; but it is far too early yet to assess its place, if any, in the long-term treatment of this disease.

Some promising results have also been reported from the early treatment of syphilitic deafness by the use of ampicillin combined with steroids.

There are two other conditions in which a growing number of reports are appearing of the successful preservation or restoration of hearing in cases of sensori-neural deafness. These are Menière's disease and some of those cases of sudden hearing loss in which the cause is obscure. In both instances the deafness is thought, by some, to be due to vascular occlusion; and in both, attempts may be made to maintain or improve the hearing by restoring an adequate blood supply to the inner ear.

Menière's disease is most commonly unilateral, and the symptoms can often be controlled by the use of vasodilator drugs (such as nicotinic acid) and labyrinthine sedatives, combined with reassurance. But in a relatively small proportion of cases, the condition may prove resistant to all such conservative medical measures; and other methods of treatment may then have to be considered.

For many years, the accepted treatment of these resistant cases was by total surgical destruction of the inner ear; but inevitably this produced total deafness in the affected ear. This was acceptable, perhaps, in unilateral cases—which most of them were—but certainly not acceptable in bilateral cases; and destructive surgery is rarely performed today. Its place has been taken by a variety of procedures— both medical and surgical, in both unilateral and bilateral cases— which aim to destroy the vestibular labyrinth whilst preserving what hearing remains.

Medically, there are still those who use streptomycin in the treatment of bilateral Menière's disease, the treatment being based on the fact that this drug, even in relatively large doses, may destroy the vestibular part without affecting the cochlear part of the inner ear. However, its effects on the cochlea are unpredictable and may develop some time after the drug has been withdrawn, and there are today very few advocates of this type of treatment.

Surgically, though, there are now several procedures which may enable the operator to control the crippling attacks of vertigo with some degree of near-certainty, without adverse effects upon the hearing. These include the use of ultra-sound, which is applied to a surgically-exposed semicircular canal; decompressing or 'shunting' of the 'water-logged' endolymphatic sac; and selective section (cutting) of the vestibular division of the VIIIth cranial nerve, the cochlear division being left intact. There is no general agreement about which is the best of these surgical manoeuvres, but each has its staunch advocates.

Another operation which is rarely practised today is that of sympathectomy—based again on the theory that Menière's disease is casued by a spasm of the arteries which supply nutrition of the inner ear, and that this spasm is caused in turn by over-activity of the 'sympathetic' nerves which control the state of the arteries.

There is considerable evidence that some cases of sensori-neural deafness of sudden onset and unknown cause may also be due to an interruption, temporary or permanent, in the blood supply to the inner ear.

Moulonguet and Bouche, in 1952, described a dramatic case in which there was strong evidence that the sudden onset of deafness was due to spasm of the end-arteries. The patient was a young man who became suddenly deaf in his right ear only a few hours after he had received an injection of an 'orthobiotic' serum. Four days later an audiogram showed a hearing loss of 65 decibels, in the speech range of frequencies, in his affected ear. Tuning fork tests showed a sensori-neural deafness, and recruitment was demonstrated. On the assumption that his deafness might be due to a spasm of the small blood vessels, he was given an intravenous injection of sodium nicotinate, to dilate the vessels. This was followed by a general flushing of the skin, and three hours later the hearing returned to normal.

'Vasodilator' drugs should be given, immediately and in high dosage, in all such cases; and in the author's experience they are treated most satisfactorily by a combination of daily intravenous drips of the drug histamine, for 3 or 4 days, with the administration by mouth of nicotinic acid or buphenine hydrochloride. The histamine is given in a dosage of 4 milligrames to 1 litre of normal saline solution, at a rate just short of that required to produce a 'histamine headache' or a rise in the pulse rate; and each 'drip' usually takes between two and four hours. The nicotinic acid and buphenine hydrochloride are each given in doses of one or two tablets three times a day.

In a limited number of these cases, the results may be extremely gratifying, but the unhappy fact remains that, by the time they reach the otologist, the majority of patients with sensori-neural deafness are beyond the help of medicine or surgery.

But advances have been made and continue to be made and much research is being done into the use of 'electrode implants' into the cochlea and higher stations of the auditory nervous pathways. This is an avenue of research which should certainly be explored further and, since many of the sounds of speech are highly redundant (Fourcin), it is conceivable that such investigations may ultimately bear fruit, especially when more is known about how *little* hearing is needed for the recognition of speech sounds, rather than how much.

The value of hearing aids, even the very best of them, is limited by the very nature of the deafness (page 79). Great reliance may therefore have to be placed on lip-reading and on the slow and painstaking process of rehabilitation. But whereas it was true to say, only twenty to twenty-five years ago, that an electrical hearing aid was almost useless for people with severe sensori-neural deafness, the design of

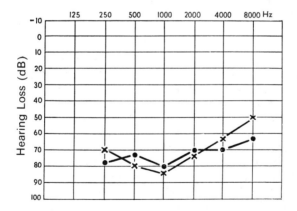

Fig. 17.8   Severe acquired sensori-neural deafness. (Pure tone audiogram).
The patient, director of a large advertising firm, became severely deaf after he had been treated with the antibiotic vancomycin, for a liver infection contracted in West Africa. He hears remarkably well with a binaural spectacle aid.

electronic apparatus has improved so enormously that more and more deafened persons, children and adults, are found to be within their range of usefulness. And no one was more agreeably surprised than I when a recent patient, who had suddenly acquired a profound deafness (Figure 17.8) in both ears after a prolonged and almost fatal illness, came back to me hearing quite remarkably well with a pair of binaural hearing-aid spectacles—regarded, until recently, as something of a plaything to be reserved solely for the use of business executives with a minor degree of conductive deafness.

18. Hysterical Deafness

The word 'Hysteria', in its true medical sense, bears little relation to the idea normally conjured up by its use in the lay mind. It has nothing to do with 'hysterical outbursts'. Correctly speaking, it is a psychogenic disturbance which may manifest itself in a wide variety of somatic (or bodily) disturbances, such as paralysis, loss of memory, loss of sensation—sometimes, but not commonly, of deafness. But there is no organic basis for the symptom, and no conscious effort to produce it. True hysteria is outside the patient's control and can usually be traced back to some unpleasant experience. It is, in fact, an unconscious escape mechanism.

Hysterical deafness is said to occur more frequently in times of war, but it was an uncommon symptom amongst British troops in action, or civilians under bombardment. Paralysis and loss of memory were much commoner manifestations of hysteria.

It is not always easy to detect the true nature of the deafness, but to one who is experienced in dealing with many deaf persons, the first (and usually an immediate) impression is that there is something rather unusual about this or that patient. At first, it is often nothing more nor less than that. There is none of that intense 'looking' for clues that is so common amongst those who have suddenly acquired severe deafness. The impression is rather that the person with hysterical deafness, although she cannot hear, does *not* look for the missing links. Instead, she tends to turn her gaze away from the speaker.

It should be kept in mind in any person who has become suddenly 'deaf' without any clear-cut predisposing cause—such as illness or injury—especially at such times of 'adjustment' or emotional stress as puberty or the menopause.

I remember very well a young girl of 13 who had become suddenly deaf nearly six months before I saw her. There was no predisposing illness or injury, and a careful history and blood tests failed to reveal any evidence or suggestion of syphilis. At the initial interview, no cause for her deafness could be found. But there was something peculiar, something not quite typical about her. Although she had been 'deaf' for six months, her voice had normal intonation and normal volume. There was no defect in it whatever. And furthermore, despite the long duration of her 'deafness', she had maintained her position at the top of her class—and she was sitting near the back!

She sat on the other side of my desk, not more than three or four feet away, and although she looked away from me throughout the interview she answered some of my questions with assurance. Yet she gave no responses at all, at any frequency and at maximum intensity, on the pure tone audiometer.

Her mother was with her and could offer no clues as to the cause of her 'deafness'. The girl was therefore referred to a teacher of the deaf, who was asked to give her intensive, frequent and regular auditory training and to repeat her audiogram at every opportunity.

By continued use of 'auditory training', through a hearing aid and reinforced by suggestion and persuasion, her audiograms improved regularly and steadily until, after less than three months, a normal audiogram was produced. And so it has remained, after several years.

Throughout the protracted course of her treatment, her story gradually unfolded. Her deafness, it appeared, had come on quite suddenly. Did she remember the occasion? Yes, she did. It happened one day at school when she was due to have her second injection against diphtheria. When first called by the school nurse, she had not answered. 'What's the matter, Jean? Are you deaf?' She returned home that day profoundly 'deaf'.

The incident may well have accounted for the particular form taken by her hysteria. But could this, in itself, be enough to account for her 'deafness' altogether? Had she any other worries? Was there anything else that she had not yet told us? There was.

Only two or three days before the onset of her 'deafness', she had been taken to the cinema by her father. And there, for the first time, she met the 'other woman'. This came as a great shock to her, for she was completely unaware that there was anything amiss between her parents. So also was her mother, and Jean was bidden not to tell her.

It was not surprising, then, that when she was offered her 'escape' a few days later, she clutched at it with open arms—probably quite unconsciously—and went home 'deaf'.

What happened to her parents, I do not know. But the girl's hearing was restored very soon after she had 'got if off her chest'.

There are several special tests, notably the Stenger test (which is described in the next chapter) which are said to be applicable to the detection of hysterical deafness, but it is my own belief that most of these tests demand a very definite conscious effort on the part of the patient, and that failure to produce responses identical with those obtained by the patient with true organic deafness is always suggestive of malingering, rather than hysteria.

True hysterical deafness is nearly always severe, often total, and usually affects both ears. It persists during sleep, but not hypnosis. And it should be treated by suggestion and persuasion, reinforced (if and when necessary) by hypnosis.

19. Feigned Deafness — Malingering

In contradistinction to true hysterical deafness, the malingerer usually feigns a deafness—commonly total—in one ear only. Malingering is a conscious act and is nearly always associated with attempts at litigation or evasion of military service. It commonly follows a genuine injury but should always be kept in mind when the word 'compensation' rears its ugly head.

Many ingenious tests have been devised for the detection of malingering, and a case report may help us to understand them.

Mr A. B., a man of 45, alleged that he had been suddenly and severely deafened by an explosion at work, and he had brought an action against his employers, who asked me to examine him on their behalf. He admitted that his hearing was normal in the right ear, but alleged that he was totally deaf in his left. Both tympanic membranes were normal and the Rinne response was positive in the right ear. But he denied hearing the tuning fork at all in the left ear, either by air conduction or by bone conduction, even when it was struck forcibly. The Weber response was referred to the right ear. This could all be quite consistent, so far, with a severe perceptive deafness in the left ear.

But when a pure tone audiogram was done, my earliest suspicions of malingering (based solely, up to that point, on his claim for compensation) were fortified. Although the audiogram showed normal hearing in the right ear, he denied hearing anything at all in his left ear, even when the testing tones were delivered at their maximum intensity (in this case 100 decibels). Now this, of course, should not happen, for even in cases of total deafness in one ear, a 'shadow' curve will be obtained, usually at a level of about 55–60 decibels (see page 43), provided that the hearing in the other ear is normal.

I therefore carried out further tests.

First of all he was asked to sit down and read a passage from a newspaper. We then put the headphones of an audiometer over his ears and asked him to go on reading. And as he was reading, a faint sound (of only 10 decibels) was introduced into his left ear—that is, the allegedly deafened ear. Immediately he raised his voice, but it returned to normal as soon as the sound was switched off. Had there been any deafness (or any severe deafness) in the left ear, this faint sound should not have been heard, and it should have had no effect on his voice. It was therefore assumed that the sound of 10 decibels was audible in the supposedly deafened ear.

The Stenger test was next performed. In this test, one delivers sounds into each ear, either separately or together, from two separate sound sources. In this case, two separate pure tone audiometers were used and the sound selected was a pure tone with a frequency of 1000 Hz. This was first delivered into his right ear (that is, the normal ear) at a level of 30 dB. He had admitted that his hearing was normal in this ear, and he now said that he could hear the testing sound.

A sound of the same frequency (1000 Hz) was then delivered into his left ear (the allegedly deafened one) from the other audiometer, while the first testing sound was still delivered continuously to the right ear. Now, had he had any deafness of the degree claimed, the introduction of this new sound (of 60 dB) into the allegedly deafened ear should not have affected his hearing for the sound delivered into his right (or normal) ear. In fact, however, he now said that he could hear nothing. Clearly the sound which he now heard in his left ear (that is, the allegedly deafened one) must have appeared louder to him than the one (of 30 dB) in his admittedly normal ear. That is to say, if he had any deafness at all in his left ear, it could not have been as severe as he had wanted us to believe; in fact, it could not have exceeded 30 decibels.

The test was repeated immediately with another sound of the same frequency (1000 Hz) but this time it was delivered into the right (normal) ear at a level of only 5 decibels. This he admitted to hearing. Another sound of the same frequency was then delivered into the left ear, at a level of 15 decibels, from the second audiometer. Once again, he denied hearing anything in either ear. Furthermore, when the earphone was removed from the left ear (the allegedly deaf one), he now denied hearing even in his right ear the sound (at 5 dB) which he had previously admitted to hearing.

Finally, he was referred to a colleague for a 'delayed speech feed-back' test. In this test, the patient is asked to read a simple text—say, from a magazine or newspaper article. As he reads this—aloud—his speech is 'fed back', through a microphone, into a special apparatus which plays it back to the patient, not *as* he says it but after a very short delay of about one-tenth of a second. He therefore hears what he has said only a fraction of a second earlier, instead of hearing what he is saying at the same moment, as we do normally.

If we are hearing what is played back after this very short delay, our speech becomes confused and slurred, and we begin to stammer —quite uncontrollably. Only rarely can conscious effort on the part of the subject stop it. And this is what happened in the present case. The patient was made to listen to the delayed speech through his allegedly damaged (left) ear, whilst the other (normal) ear was masked and so could not affect the results of the test. His speech became very markedly halting and more than normally slurred as soon as the delayed speech in his allegedly damaged (left) ear reached the intensity at which people with normal hearing exhibit the same symptoms. He must therefore have heard his own delayed speech in his left ear.

Békésy audiometry can also be helpful in such cases, and a type V tracing (Jerger) is typical of feigned deafness. The diagnosis can be further confirmed by objective tests of hearing, and cortical evoked response audiometry and electro-cochleography may be particuarly helpful in this context.

20. Some Psychological Aspects of Deafness

'Deafness is worse than blindness, so they say—it is the loneliness, the sense of isolation, that makes it so, and the lack of understanding in the minds of ordinary hearing people. The problem of the child deaf from birth . . . is quite different from that of the man or woman who has become completely deafened after school age or in adult life. The 'hard of hearing' person whose deafness has developed slowly over the years . . . is different again. But for all of them the handicap is the same—the handicap of the silent world, the difficulty of communicating with the hearing and speaking world.'

These are the words of Scott Stevenson. This is deafness in a nutshell. Whatever its cause, whenever its onset, whatever its degree, the most conspicuous handicap of deafness—at any age—is the difficulty experienced by the deaf in communicating with the hearing, and by the hearing with the deaf.

The deaf poet David Wright, in his fascinating 'personal account' of deafness, expresses the generous view that 'it is the non-deaf who absorb a large part of the impact of the disability. The limitations imposed by deafness,' he says, 'are often less noticed by its victims than by those with whom they have to do' . . . 'Having to dispense with the easy exchange of trivialities which is the oil to the wheels of conversation and to the business of living,' he adds is 'an undramatic but not minor disadvantage of deafness, felt less positively by the deaf than by their hearing friends.'

The deaf child

Michael Reed has emphasized that the child who is born deaf, or the child who has acquired deafness early in life, is subject to all the frustrations of the hearing child. But to these is added the further frustration of his inability to communicate with his family and friends by the quickest method possible—speech. As long as his deafness goes unnoticed, his frustrations are exaggerated, his temper tantrums worse. This can be minimized only by the early recognition of his handicap.

One of the greatest needs of any child is security, but this need is not so easily met in the case of the deaf child. 'During the months before the (normal) baby can crawl,' says Michael Reed, 'much of his time is spent in a pram or cot, lying sleeping or perhaps idly playing with rattles. Sometimes he becomes fretful. He may be uncomfortable or a little afraid. Usually his mother will soothe him from a distance by gentle comforting sounds. Baby becomes happier and often settles down. The deaf baby cannot hear these sounds of comfort coming from a distance. His whimpers become wails. If one knows that the baby is deaf, the situation is still under control. Instead of comforting by sounds from a distance one can move into the baby's line of vision. Often all that is necessary is that baby should be aware of the presence of his mother.'

The intellectual as well as the emotional development of the deaf child is handicapped by his lack of speech, since thoughts depend a great deal on words for their expression. This was emphasized by L. Gardner, educational psychologist at the Hospital for Sick Children, in Great Ormond Street. 'It is difficult,' he wrote, 'to think without words, and without words the deaf child cannot easily share the thoughts and experiences of other people and thereby further his intellectual development.'

No less important are the psychological repercussions on the parents of a deaf child. To quote once again from Michael Reed: 'some may feel resentful, others guilty. Some terribly apprehensive of the future, others quite bewildered, and a few who refuse to believe it. . . . No one can hope to help their child fully while these feelings remain. There is no guilt. There must be no fear. The fact that there is deafness must be accepted. There must be no resentment. All these feelings put a brake on progress.'

There can be no doubt that one of the greatest difficulties facing the parents of a deaf child is their acceptance of his handicap. It is always tragic to see the bewilderment of a mother who is seeking a second, or a third, or even a tenth opinion—in the hope that someone sooner or later, will tell her that her child is *not* deaf—only to be told once again, in most cases, that he is. Deafness *must* be accepted. The task that lies ahead is often very great, but it cannot be properly begun until one has succeeded in removing the enormous psychological barrier of non-acceptance. Nor can there be any let-up. The task is never-ending, and it must continue, all through the school years, right up to adolescence and on into adult life.

'It is not normal to be deaf', wrote Gesell in 1956, but the deaf can be remarkably normal as individual personalities if we guide them into the right methods of managing their handicap. Our aim should be to convert the deaf child not into a somewhat fictitious version of a normal hearing child, but into a well-adjusted non-hearing child who is completely managing the limitations of his sensory defect.

The school years

Two of the greatest problems facing the deaf child are his education, and his integration into the society of his hearing peers.

Dr Robert Thouless, Reader in Educational Psychology in the University of Cambridge, has spoken thus of these vexed problems: 'There is no disagreement as to what is desired for the handicapped child. We all agree that he must be given the best *education* available . . . by teachers trained in methods of imparting knowledge and skills, in ways that get past the obstacles presented by the child's handicap. It is also agreed, though perhaps less emphatically, that the handicapped child must be given the best opportunity for *social development*. This means the opportunity of taking his place in the world in general and not merely amongst a group of similarly handicapped people'.

'The difficulties that arise are largely due to the possibility of these two aims being in conflict. The most efficient methods of education may be those that do not best contribute to normal social development. The aim of creating conditions for normal social development may be one that makes less easy the special type of education suitable for the handicapped.'

Solely oral education is, of course, essential to the ultimate integration of deaf children into the general society of hearing adults; but there is an opposing view which, whilst applauding this goal, believes nevertheless that it can be achieved to only a limited extent by the majority of deaf persons. According to this latter philosophy, manualism is permissible in addition to oralism. 'A well-integrated, happy deaf individual' is preferred to 'a pale imitation of a hearing person' (Quigley).

In discussing the *educational* advantages of segregation, Dr Thouless argues that, if a group of handicapped children are educated together, it is possible to have teachers skilled in the methods of overcoming the handicap, and also to provide any apparatus that may be necessary for the special methods of teaching employed; that segregated education may remove the sense of discouragement which might afflict the handicapped child in the surroundings of an ordinary school; and that it may reduce the harmful psychological effect of over-protection of the handicapped child by his parents.

But, he admits, we must not lose sight of the socio-psychological *dis*advantages of segregation. 'The handicapped child,' he says, 'growing up in a group of other handicapped children, is learning to adapt himself to a society of people suffering from similar handicaps, and not to one composed of normal people. This is perhaps more true of deaf children than of other types of handicapped children, because living with other deaf children may encourage them to develop methods of communication which are adapted only to other deaf and not to normal people.'

This point has also been emphasized by Pierre Gorman, himself born profoundly deaf. 'In the United Kingdom,' he writes, 'practically all deaf children go to special schools taking in only deaf children'— in this context, he refers only to those children who are *profoundly* deaf from birth or shortly afterwards—'The normal adults who are most in contact with them are teachers who have recieved professional training to understand *in a particular way* the psychological and educational needs of their deaf pupils. As a result, a protected climate is set up, and the teachers become regarded as typical normal persons owing to the limited opportunities available to the children for making outside contacts with other members of the community . . . This restricted and constant contact with certain normal adults (i.e. the teachers) in a very limited environment tends to make the child think that persons outside school will behave in the same way as the teachers do towards him. The possibility that people outside this closed environment often behave in a contrary way may never occur to him.'

The deaf adolescent

Adolescence is never an easy time. It is much less easy for the *deaf* adolescent, who still finds it a difficult time even if he is not prelingually deaf and he has good speech. Deafness accentuates the problems of adolescence in relation to sexual maturity, to seeking a job and perhaps to leaving home; and as a result, there is a high incidence of emotional disturbance among deaf adolescents.

The most striking thing about the average school-leaver from a school for the deaf is his difficulty in communicating with most hearing people. Those who integrate with the hearing community usually have a useful degree of residual hearing.

To the general problems of adolescence, the deaf-school leaver must therefore add his own special problem of integration into normal hearing society. But the success or failure of this integration will depend, at least in part, on the attitude towards him of the hearing people whom he meets.

Many fail to integrate and need to be introduced to the world of other deaf adolescents and of deaf adults, by social workers who complain that the schools have failed to prepare them properly for integration with the community of the hearing. And so they seek the company of other deaf youths—in the clubs and in the missions. At present, this seems to be the inevitable course for some, indeed for many of those adolescents who are profoundly deaf. It is their only means of social intercourse. Nor is this to say that it should be otherwise. But it is an issue of vital importance, and it has even been said that this should be the central theme of the whole educational system for deaf children.

According to Mervin Garretson, there is a fairly large proportion of deaf school-leavers who withdraw from hearing society into the relatively small and restricted ('though safe') place provided by organizations and societies for the deaf and hard-of-hearing. They thus escape the feeling of being 'left out'; they reject, and are rejected by, hearing society.

At the other extreme, there are those who reject the world of the deaf and spend their lives aspiring to be acceptable in the normally hearing world. They find themselves in the 'no-man's-land' between the world which they themselves have rejected and the way of life which they desire but which rejects them.

Between these two extremes, according to Garretson, are the great majority of school-leavers who believe that they have learned to accept the realities of deafness. Recognizing that they belong to a 'marginal' group, they ask their hearing friends to accept them as deaf persons, and they tend to seek interests in which hearing is not too significant a factor.

The second most obvious thing about the average deaf school leaver is his linguistic and educational retardation, and apart from the difficulties of social and emotional adjustment, he must also face the difficulties of vocational adjustment. Rainer and Altshuler found, in New York, that 30 per cent of school-leavers interviewed by them had no vocational plans at all at the time they left school. Only 40 per cent felt that their school training had been at all helpful in enabling them to obtain employment. The vast majority performed some form of manual labour, but more than half of these became skilled workers.

There is great need for a systematic approach to the vocational guidance of the deaf.

The deafened adult

The psychological problems of the adult who has become deafened, slowly or suddenly, after he has left school, presents quite a different picture. True it is that his main handicap is still one of communication. But he has learnt to speak. He has grown up in a speaking society—and he knows no other. Now he is isolated, cut off. More and more he will tend to avoid company until, if active measures are not taken to overcome his handicap, he will turn to the life of a recluse. To stress —the normal stress of everyday life—is added strain.

'A man who does not hear well has to listen,' said the late F. W. Watkyn-Thomas. 'Few people speak clearly and distinctly. With normal hearing a great deal must be subconsciously guessed or supplied from the context; perfect hearing finds difficulty with gabblers and voice-droppers. A deaf man misses much more, and so he has to supply much more from the imperfectly heard context. Even in casual conversation, he has to *listen*—a voluntary action which means attention and concentration, and so a varying but ever-present degree of strain'.

'This element of strain is constant in the make-up of deafness. . . . It is important for the patient as well as for his deafness. It goes some way to account for the irritability of the deaf; but here we must make allowance for ageing arteries and perhaps for natural annoyance with imperfect elocution.'

But Watkyn-Thomas, who was himself hard-of-hearing, was writing only about lesser degrees of hearing loss; and there is much more to it than that.

In a recent symposium on the rehabilitation of the adult deaf, held at the Royal Society of Medicine in London in 1975, Wendy Galbraith said this: 'Psychologically an acquired hearing loss brings an inevitable deterioration in the individual's security and self-esteem. He loses touch with his environment from which, as a normally hearing person, he gained much information. Where hearing is an essential for the continuation of a job, a deafened person may have to take up an alternative occupation and this is likely to be of an inferior nature to that held previously; this may well produce a sense of failure'.

And in the same symposium, Dr John Brothwood reminded us that we are concerned with a wide range of understandable reactions to persistent and severe deafness, the recognition of which is all important in the management of the deaf person's handicap. 'This', he said, 'includes maladaptive behaviour, the first sign of which may be difficulty in coping with everyday life, followed by . . . social withdrawal. In turn this may lead to depressive illness, which is so common among the deaf, or more rarely to the development of paranoid states . . . There are, of course, many other handicaps of a less serious nature . . . which may arise in the course of severe and persistent deafness, such as apparent inattention . . . which may be misinterpreted as obtuseness, eccentricity (or) confusion'.

Nowhere are these effects more apparent than in the adult who has become deafened *suddenly*, and Miss Rosemary McCall, Director of the Link Centre for Deafened People in Eastbourne, has written that 'Because communication is the prime element of all social life, deafness is a social disaster which profoundly affects not only the deafened person but also his family and everyone who meets him'; and amongst the less obvious, more subtle and insidious effects of deafness, she names (amongst others) the need for adjustment to a soundless environment; the disturbance of not being able to hear one's own voice; the embarrassment of misunderstandings; the uncertainty created when people act unexpectedly without explanation; and the constant alertness needed for communication, which is very demanding.

As one of her guests once commented: 'Deafness cannot do other than destroy the very basis of self-confidence'; and when Jack Ashley was confronted suddenly with total deafness, he described it as 'like drowning in a sea of silence'. To which Miss McCall adds this very perceptive comment: 'A drowning man does not want sympathy or research—he wants a life line.' And this is where rehabilitation begins.

21. Rehabilitation of the Deaf

The last few years have witnessed an enormous upsurge of interest in the rehabilitation of the deaf, and it can be no accident that the growing awareness and concern of successive governments has followed or coincided with the tragic experience of that well-known politician, Mr Jack Ashley, C.H., Member of Parliament for Stoke-on-Trent. Himself deafened suddenly in 1967, he has poured his apparently inexhaustible energies into improving the lot of all handicapped persons, and the years that have passed since the last edition of this monograph have seen the setting up of a number of bodies to consider the welfare and rehabilitation of the deaf of all ages.

Misleading advertisements for commerical hearing aids have become far less frequent since the institution of the industry's own ethical body—the Hearing Aid Industry Association—and of the Hearing Aid Council, set up in 1968 by an Act of Parliament. The Medical Research Council has recently set up two Working Parties, one of them concerned exclusively with research needs for rehabilitation of the deaf; its final report is being drawn up at the time of writing. The Department of Health and Social Security (DHSS) has appointed an Advisory Committee on Services for Hearing Impaired People whose membership has a very broad spectrum of representation from the professions of medicine, audiology, nursing, education and the physical and social sciences, as well as technical and voluntary services. Representatives from the DHSS have also visited several of the Scandinavian countries, where services for the deaf are very highly developed, and they have produced a comprehensive but confidential report of those visits, as well as an individual report (the Rawson report) which has received wide circulation and some (unjustified) criticism.

The British Association of Otolaryngologists has conducted a survey into the rehabilitative requirements of the deafened adult, until recently a relatively neglected member of the deaf population; and a similar investigation is being undertaken by the Department of Applied Social Studies in the Polytechnic of North London. The deaf adult is also receiving special attention at the City Literary Institute in London. The Link Centre in Eastbourne, which was registered as a charity in 1972, holds residential courses for adults who have become suddenly deafened; and the British Broadcasting Corporation has recently shown a series of ten weekly programmes on television under the title of 'I see what you mean'.

But perhaps the most significant advance in this direction is the recognition by the Department of Health of a new type of specialist, the consultant audiological physician, who shall have the future over-all responsibility for rehabilitation of the deaf of all ages and for organisation of the necessary services.

These are, indeed, great and significant strides in the right direction, and it is to be hoped that the recommendations made by these many new committees and reports will be implemented as soon as funds become available.

Where, then, does rehabilitation begin? It begins when medical or surgical treatment has failed, or has proved to be impossible.

The main purpose of rehabilitation of the deaf is to overcome the handicap. Or, in the words of Wendy Galbraith, 'the aim . . . must initially be to help him come to terms with the handicap and to develop skills which will alleviate the adverse results of deafness so that he can continue to function within his social and occupational competency'.

Hearing aids can help the majority of deaf people, whether they have been born deaf or become deafened. But no aid should ever be issued without a thorough explanation of its uses and limitations, its working and its maintenance. The simple provision of one of these instruments is not sufficient to produce a return to normality, and experience has shown that, after an initial period of euphoria (when the patient finds that he can hear sounds again), a period of·depression all too often follows when he realizes that many of the sounds that he hears are too distorted for instant recognition; and in many instances, auditory training is an essential supplement to the aid, both in children and in adults, and there is no doubt that better progress can be made when a 'hearing therapist' can see the patient regularly, to help him to come to terms with his handicap and to make the best use of his hearing aid.

Unfortunately auditory training, although more or less available to most deaf children in the United Kingdom, is often very difficult to obtain for adults. In some countries, auditory training is given almost routinely to virtually every person who is provided with a hearing aid and, although one might doubt the necessity for such intensive therapy in all cases, there is little doubt that the deafened adult in this country is poorly catered for by comparison. It is not surprising that even simple follow-up with hearing aids is poor, and that all too often only very basic instruction is provided, when one realizes that approximately 65 000 of these instruments are fitted every year in Great Britain, by no more than 250 audiology technicians, who are responsible also for most of the audiometry. And although theoretically, rehabilitative facilities are supposed to be available through local education authorities, social service departments and departments of employment, the hearing therapist is a luxury so far confined to a limited number of the larger cities and towns.

In the recent survey conducted by the British Association of Otolaryngologists, it was estimated that about one in every four adults deafened by sensori-neural hearing loss is likely to require the services of a hearing therapist; and this estimate would tend to be confirmed by experience in those European countries where rehabilitative services are well developed and where it has been suggested that 20 to 25 per cent of all such persons require auditory training, lip-reading tuition and exercises in speech preservation.

There are very few deaf persons, whatever their age and whatever the degree of their hearing loss, who cannot 'hear' better when they can see the speaker. In many instances, the ability to lip-read is acquired spontaneously; in some a truly remarkable facility is developed. But there are few deaf children, or adults, who cannot derive some benefit from formal instruction in lip-reading; yet lip-reading facilities are poorly distributed within the United Kingdom, and in some areas they are virtually non-existent.

There are, of course, some notable exceptions to this statement, and in London and the Home Counties, for instance, such facilities are fairly readily available. And for those who are suddenly plunged into the despondency of deafness ('drowning in a sea of silence', as Jack Ashley puts it), there is the Link Centre, which provides (not only for the subject himself but also for his family) 'adjustment to a soundless environment'. It aims 'to give comfort, courage and fresh hope'; 'to provide guidelines for the future'; and 'to draw people together, professionals, deafened people and their families, to form a basis for further progress in understanding'.

Speech correction is another important aspect of rehabilitation, and no programme of rehabilitation can be considered complete without attention to it. Several years ago, a research project was initiated at University College in London, under the direction of Dr Adrian Fourcin, to investigate ways in which the 'laryngograph' can help deaf adults and children to improve their speech; and it has been found that it can help deaf persons with control of the pitch register, with the acquisition and control of pitch changes, with timing and with voicing.

We must not forget, however, that not every deaf person can be taught to communicate by speech and we cannot ignore the many children leaving our schools for the deaf without recognizable speech; nor can we ignore those many other deaf persons, including a number of deaf adults who, for a variety of reasons, are unable to communicate by speech. These latter include a small number of persons who have become deafened long after speech has developed, but who nevertheless prefer a non-oral means of communication; and the rehabilitation of this relatively small group of the deaf community must therefore include manual methods, however simple or complex, as the sole or a supplementary means of language development. Such methods include *sign language* (in which the signs are based on ideas or pictures, rather than on words) or *finger-spelling* (in which a visible symbol represents each letter of the alphabet, and words are simply spelt out letter by letter). *Cued speech* gives a manual indication of the sounds of speech; unlike finger-spelling, it is based on phonetics and it may therefore reinforce lip-reading and speech. It has been defined as 'a method of communication in which eight configurations and four positions of one (either) hand are used to supplement the visible manifestations of natural speech'. The *Danish hand-mouth system* is also phonetic and is used in conjunction with lip-reading; only the consonant sounds are indicated by the hand and, being also phonetic, it reinforces speech and lip-reading. *The Paget-Gorman Systematic Sign System* is a grammatical form of signing in which each word is indicated.

It would be impossible to over-emphasize the importance of the part played by the family, friends and working colleagues of the deaf in their general rehabilitation. 'If they can be persuaded to speak clearly, to avoid shouting, and to exercise patience', wrote the late F.W. Watkyn-Thomas, 'a common source of friction is eliminated. But the patient must do his share; for one thing, he must be careful to speak clearly himself, and not perpetuate the speech errors of which he complains in others. Also, if people take the trouble to speak clearly to him, he must encourage them by taking the trouble to listen. On such elementary points as these does a great deal of a patient's rehabilitation depend.' To this, it should be added that most deaf persons find it much easier to follow a spoken conversation if they know what is being talked about. It is therefore always helpful to warn a deaf friend when a new subject is going to be discussed. Furthermore, he may miss several sentences in their entirety and may find it no easier to hear the same words if they are repeated. When it is clear that a deaf person has not understood, or has mis-understood, such a sentence, it is helpful to re-phrase it and to express it with quite a different choice of words.

There is a great need for the further development of social services for the deaf. Essentially, social service departments, as at present constituted, are multi-service organizations, and they have statutory responsibility for a very wide range of social problems involving citizens of all ages and of widely differing walks in life; and whilst most social workers would agree that they should all have *some* basic knowledge and understanding of deafness, there is at present little provision for training them in the various aspects of the handicap. However, there are likely soon to be new developments in the special training of such workers in the management of handicaps, including deafness.

Far too many employers still tend to underestimate the capabilities of the deaf, whether the employee has been born with his handicap or has acquired it, and experience has shown that a capable deaf person is almost always under-employed. This may not be so at the unskilled level, but at the semi-skilled level and certainly at the skilled level, it *is* so. The acknowledged jobs for children who have left special schools for the deaf are still too menial-machinists' jobs for girls, with skilled or unskilled labouring jobs for boys. There are, it is true, a few clerical appointments for girls, including jobs as comptometer operators and copy typists, and there is an increasing number of boys entering the trades; but still many deaf-school leavers are capable of much better jobs than they have. That this should be so is due largely to a lack of facilities for the very deaf school leaver to be trained; to the delays which he may have to accept before employment when such further training *is* possible; and perhaps above all, to the unsympathetic attitude of employers.

However competent a deaf person may be, communication in-evitably is slower, and few employers are prepared to accept this. If deaf persons are ever to reach levels of employment which are commensurate with their abilities, then more special training must be available and they should be encouraged to train for technical or technological work in which oral communication need only be minimal.

It may be beneficial for a deaf person to register under the Disabled Person's Employment Acts, and the Disablement Resettlement Officer at any local Employment Exchange can provide helpful advice. There are almost a hundred special training units of various kinds in the United Kingdom, and many of them are suitable for hearing-impaired people. There is a residential college in Durham which is especially suitable for profoundly deaf persons, with or without speech; and the Royal National Institute for the Deaf has its own residential hostel at Newton Abbot for maladjusted deaf youths.

There is an urgent need for many more audiology technicians—there always has been; and there is a desperately urgent need for hearing therapists. Initially they are likely to be drawn from workers for the deaf in many different fields, but outside these fields there is little doubt that experience in teaching would be an invaluable asset to new recruits. From whatever section of the community they are drawn, extra training will certainly be necessary; for whoever works as a hearing therapist must understand the effects of the handicap, the working and limitations of individual and environmental aids to hearing, the principles and techniques of visual communication (including lip-speaking), and the attitudes of hearing society to what Dr Samuel Johnson described as 'the most desperate of human calamities'.

22. Tinnitus

'Tinnitus' is the name given to a sensation of sound in one or both ears, and it is a very common accompaniment to deafness.

Many sufferers from tinnitus are barely conscious of its presence; others are driven to desperation with it. It is, indeed, a most distressing symptom to some persons, and it may be the only complaint in many.

Although research has been, and continues to be, conducted into the symptom of tinnitus, there is at present little that can be done to relieve it and its mechanism is but little understood. Nevertheless, there are certain facts about tinnitus which may provide at least a working hypothesis about its origin.

In the first place, *when tinnitus is present, there is nearly always some hearing loss.* This is not to say that every patient who complains of tinnitus, will also complain of deafness; and in practice many patients who suffer from tinnitus are unaware of any difficulty in hearing, at least for conversation. But if a pure-tone audiogram is done in every patient—and it should *always* be done in persons suffering from tinnitus—it is extremely rare, in my experience, to find absolutely normal hearing, the commonest finding being that of a high frequency hearing loss, often at 4000 or 6000 Hz, and often so slight in degree as to cause little or no difficulty with conversation. It may, however, be a warning of impending deafness and it is seen, for example, in those who shoot, long before there is any consciousness of difficulty in hearing.

Conversely, *when there is no measurable hearing loss, there is rarely any tinnitus.* In other words, the person who has absolutely normal hearing, very rarely complains of tinnitus. Why should this be? It is my belief that every one of us is born with noises in the head. They are there from birth to death. Why, then, are we not conscious of them when our hearing is normal? In my view, it is because there is no such thing as complete silence in everyday life—not even in the heart of the country, in the still of the night. Even under these circumstances, a sensitive sound level meter will measure *some* ambient noise— perhaps 20 dB, perhaps 25 or 30 dB. And provided that our hearing is normal, this faint ambient noise will be sufficient to over-shadow (or 'mask') our own intrinsic head noises—generated, possibly, by blood rushing through the vessels—large and small—within the head.

I have twice been in an 'anechoic chamber', which is near to silence, and within a minute of two of closing the door to all external sounds,

I have become conscious of a faint noise in both ears which I can only describe as the sort of sound that I used to hear, as a boy, when I held a sea-shell to my ear on a beach and heard the echoes of wind and waves. This is 'white noise' (see page 19); and so is ambient noise when all is quiet.

Furthermore sometimes, when I am tried and I bury my head in a pillow, I am conscious—in the buried ear—of my own pulse, this is noticed by many people, especially after physical or emotional stress, when the pulse is more rapid and 'bounding'.

We all have noise in the head. Ah, you may say, but this is 'white' noise, mine is not. I hear a high whistle, like the sound emitted by a whistling kettle or an old steam train; or others will say: but the sound *I* hear is like a low buzzing or rumbling. To which I would reply that, generally speaking, *the pitch of a subjective tinnitus nearly always coincides with the frequency of the maximal hearing loss.* Several years ago, my friend Ellis Douek, then working at the Royal Free Hospital and now an eminent otologist at Guy's Hospital in London, published a paper with Joy Reid, a highly skilled and experienced audiology technician, on 'Tinnitus Pitch'. And they found that, if the pitch of a patient's tinnitus is compared with the frequencies of a pure-tone audiometer, it is nearly always found that the pitch of the tinnitus approximates most closely to the frequency of the maximal hearing loss: so that, for example, if the hearing loss is greatest in the high frequencies (as in acoustic trauma), so the tinnitus is usually high-pitched; and if the loss is maximal in the low frequencies (as in most cases of early Menière's disease), so the tinnitus is usually low-pitched.

So what?, you may ask. And I would reply as follows: We all have 'white' noise in our heads. There is always 'white' noise in the 'atmosphere'. If your hearing is defective in the high frequencies, you will not hear the high frequencies—either consciously or unconsciously—within the spectrum of 'white' background noises; but you will still hear the high frequencies within the spectrum of your own intrinsic 'white' noise, for this is not masked by the (inaudible) high-tones in ambient sound.

Then why don't you hear these noises when the hearing is normal? Because the intensity of ambient noise, in the normal conditions of everyday life is *just* sufficiently greater than the intensity of our intrinsic head noises. A lot of work has been done on this aspect of tinnitus, and it is an interesting fact that *tinnitus can usually be abolished by ambient noise.* If, for example, someone suffers from tinnitus which has a frequency of 4000 Hz, this can usually be abolished by introducing into the affected ear (from an audiometer) a sound of the same frequency; and the point at which the tinnitus disappears will usually be found to be not more than 30 or 35 dB above the threshold of hearing at that particular frequency.

It is well known that tinnitus is usually much more noticeable in quiet than in noisy surroundings (although it may be made temporarily worse by exposure to excessively loud traffic and other noises); and many sufferers from tinnitus are helped by 'bathing' their surroundings in the sounds of a radio, or even by amplifying background noises with a hearing aid—provided, of course, that there is useful and usable residual hearing.

Furthermore, *tinnitus can often be reduced or abolished by the restoration of normal or near-normal hearing,* by Nature, or by medical or surgical measures, as for instance, after a successful stapedectomy in a patient with deafness and tinnitus due to otosclerosis; and in one recent series of cases, the incidence of tinnitus was reduced by surgery from one-in-three to only one-in-ten.

But surely, tinnitus is a sensation of sound, and all sensations of sound are carried to the brain by the auditory nerve? True. So, in those cases when the hearing cannot be restored, why can't you cut the auditory nerve and abolish the tinnitus that way? The answer to that is that hearing is a perceptual process, which takes place in the brain; and when the sensations of sound have reached the brain, countless numbers of times, not even cutting off the supply of renewed impulses will necessarily abolish those sensations altogether. I have never heard a child *born* deaf complaining of tinnitus. Nerve section sometimes works, but the operation is a major one and it is not by any means always successful. Occasionally it may alter the nature of a tinnitus; more often than not, it will remain the same. It is rather like the symptoms of a 'phantom limb', experienced by those who have had to have a limb amputated; long after such an event, the patient may still experience the sensations of his big toe turning up or down, for example—sensations which can be, and often are, recalled for the remainder of his life.

Such an hypothesis as I have developed makes no pretence to explain the sudden, short-lived, piercing, screeching tinnitus which affects so many adults—fortunately, only for a few seconds usually—from time to time; nor does it explain in any way those rare cases of 'objective' tinnitus, in which noises can be heard, not only by the patient, but by other listeners. It takes no account of those hallucinations of voices or other sounds which are of psychogenic origin; and it ignores those tuneful or rythmical sounds which may be indicative of temporal lobe epilepsy. But it does attempt to provide some sort of an explanation of that type of tinnitus with which the otologist is most commonly confronted; and it does attempt to provide some sort of a basis for the explanation and re-assurance which play such an essential part in the management of this difficulty problem.

Is it dangerous? By itself, never. But it may be the first symptom of an acoustic neuroma, and this condition should always be excluded, especially in cases of unilateral tinnitus, if there is any reason at all to suspect such a diagnosis.

Hypertension (high blood pressure) is a relatively uncommon cause which is easy to exclude, and a general medical check is never out of place.

In those cases (the vast majority) in which there is an associated hearing loss, advice should be given about ways and means of preventing further loss: for example, in cases of acoustic trauma due to shooting, protective devices should always be worn during future exposures; and in cases of ototoxicity, the offending drug should be withdrawn immediately if a satisfactory alternative exists.

Drugs are rarely useful in controlling this symptom. Too often they are both ineffective and depressing and the use of tranquillizers is rarely to be advised. Almost the only exception to this general 'rule' is the occasional prescription of a simple sedative for those surprisingly few cases in which the tinnitus prevents sleep—with inevitable tiredness, which usually makes it worse.

In a recent article in *The Guardian,* Charles Mandell, secretary of the British Association of the Hard of Hearing, himself a sufferer for forty years, was quoted as saying this: 'The best way to treat tinnitus is the same as one treats the club bore. You accept you must listen to him and do it with the best grace you can. So if head noises are unduly loud, to listen to them makes them acceptable as much as anything can; and trying to put them out of one's mind, being impossible, is a useless waste of emotion'.

Regrettably, there is little more that the present sufferer can do about it; but it is conceivable that developments in electronics may hold out some hope of future relief of this symptom, especially if efforts are concentrated on the more precise assessment of tinnitus pitch.

Appendix I. Testing Materials for Use in Audiology Clinics

PLASTIC BEAKERS, RINGS AND TOY DRUMS
Obtainable from
  Paul and Marjorie Abbatt Toys Ltd.,
    Toys and Nursery Equipment,
      74, Wimpole Street,
        LONDON, W.I. 01-487 4382

XYLOPHONE BARS—(Frequencies of 500, 1000, 2000 and 4000 Hz)
Obtainable from:
  Boosey and Hawkes Ltd.,
    Musical Instruments,
      295, Regent Street,
        LONDON, W.I. 01-580 2060

PITCH PIPES—(Several frequencies, including the 'speech frequencies'
  above)
Obtainable from:
  R. F. Stevens Ltd.,
    Reed Organ Builders,
      9, Leighton Place,
        LONDON, N.W.5. 01-485 2745

MUSICAL BOXES—'SPIN' RATTLES
Obtainable from:
  Hamleys of Regent Street Ltd.,
    Toys, Sports and Games,
      200, Regent Street,
        LONDON, W.I. 01-734 3161

HIGH—FREQUENCY RATTLES
Obtainable from:
  Department of Audiology and Education of the Deaf,
    The University,
      MANCHESTER, M 13 9PL

TUNING FORKS—(Complete range of frequencies, in C scale)
Obtainable from:
  Down Bros. and Mayer and Phelps Ltd.,
    Surgical Instrument Manufacturers,
      34, New Cavendish Street,
        LONDON, W.I. 01-486 3611

Acoustic Tiles—(for the sound insulation of testing rooms)
Obtainable from:
> Anderson Construction Company Ltd.,
>> Clifton House,
>>> Euston Road,
>>>> LONDON, N.W.1. 01-387 7465

'Stycar' Test Material—(for screening tests in infants)
Obtainable from:
> The National Foundation for Educational Research in England and Wales,
>> The Mere,
>>> Upton Park,
>>>> SLOUGH, BUCKINGHAMSHIRE.

Appendix II.   Words and Sentence Lists

List 1 (Monosyllabic Words)	*List* 2 (Bisyllabic Words)
1. Glove	1. Balloon
2. Flag	2. Playground
3. Mouse	3. Bagpipe
4. Flame	4. Eyebrow
5. Pup	5. Grandson
6. Map	6. Cowboy
7. Cow	7. Orange
8. Five	8. Moonlight
9. Eyes	9. Toothbrush
10. Feet	10. Facecloth
11. Mop	11. Platform
12. Soap	12. Teatime
13. Patch	13. Toilet
14. Smash	14. Sunshine
15. Sheep	15. Picture
16. Kite	16. Colour
17. Leg	17. Pancake
18. Chicks	18. Doormat
19. Bone	19. Bellows
20. Egg	20. Shadow
21. Knee	
22. Star	
23. Shade	
24. Pump	
25. Ink	

WORD LISTS FOR SPEECH AUDIOMETRY

List 1

Cut	Now	Lid	Heard	Men	Hut.	Choice
Sin	Jam	Deaf	Raw	Wish	Ten	Veal
Bite	Wrong	Yard	Tin	Ton	Less	There
Will	Near	Pays	Right	Good	Face	Move
Bone	Keys	White	Sack	Dip	So	Thick

List 2

Tap	Nil	Gun	Comb	None	Song	Yet
Chair	Sit	Pet	Lid	Term	Nor	Boy
Bud	Laugh	Line	Mile	Wait	With	Row
Shed	Rear	Van	Den	Take	Sick	Suit
Juice	Hose	Weave	Side	Thief	Rick	His

List 3

Cat	Nose	Wool	Sight	Can	Said	Guard
Thing	Nib	Hen	Dish	Them	Luck	Wit
Tip	Team	Save	Nought	Yes	Rail	Rough
Beer	Kid	Toy	Dodge	Wise	Fuss	Chill
Verse	Tea	Rope	Nine	Dare	Moon	How

List 4

Boot	Bough	Sieve	Fierce	Then	Wick	Learn
Roe	Need	Yell	Could	Miss	Chat	Run
Wig	Wedge	Dumb	High	Poise	Tack	Not
Raid	Hair	Pass	Thin	Sing	Vote	Shine
Says	Lay	Feed	Kill	Mud	Torn	Tight

List 5

Note	Fun	Thought	Ride	While	Rut	Had
Dig	That	Cease	Vow	Tier	Led	Cave
Died	Shoes	Run	Gin	Toys	Firm	Set
Mess	Long	Nip	Well	Bear	Soap	Him
Rook	Say	Key	Yarn	Tick	Win	Chin

List 6

Cock	Pain	Cheese	Hush	Wed	Wing	Doubt
Sigh	Voice	Red	Ridge	Man	Dear	Nice
This	Born	Thud	Rude	Keen	Sag	Low
Care	Limb	Net	May	Sole	Fit	Fight
Whizz	Love	Yacht	Hip	Turn	Bet	Tar

List 7

Tan	Wear	Yawn	Let	Ray	Jut	Fear
Room	Feet	Till	Hark	Vice	Bell	No
Town	Done	Ship	Ring	Sat	Thumb	Niece
Wood	Those	Sir	Coin	Ditch	Made	Guess
Kick	Sign	Bit	Dive	Was	Lip	Head

List 8

Bid	Tell	Mug	Gnat	Bin	Neat	Third
Dark	Wet	Hang	Worn	Mouse	Toe	Rim
Fed	Way	Live	Loss	Theirs	Tiers	Took

Vine	Nut	Seek	Pill	Fish	Such	Race
Dough	You	Join	Kiss	Rye	Hid	Pen

List 9

Cow	Vase	Pan	Rib	Dim	Year	Course
Lit	Soil	Rid	Fig	Known	Should	When
Woke	Sap	Bus	Hung	My	Sun	Met
Teach	Root	Night	Live (Liv)	Dares	They	Deck
Wade	Hit	Toss	Jet	Thigh	Kneel	Fern

List 10

Ran	Wren	Which	Loud	Thaw	Do	Give
But	Fan	Harm	Knit	Joy	Debt	Though
Bed	King	Wine	Seed	Din	Case	Rip
Sum	Tail	Week	Mice	Five	Hook	Shut
Pin	Low	Tot	Years	Tears (Tares)	Nurse	Sell

SENTENCE LISTS FOR LIVE VOICE TESTS

List 1

The boy found a penny
Mother cut some bread
The kitten drank its milk
The girl lost her doll
I had a cup of tea
The fish is in the water
She sat by the fire
The plate is on the table
David went to the park
I paddled in the sea
The cat caught a moth
The boys sailed their boats on the pond
He saw some flowers
They went to the seaside
She made sand castles
I paddled in the sea
Jack fell in the water
You had cake for tea
The birds flew over the river

Susie had some cake
The baby cried
Freddie washed his face
The dog bit the cat
Daddy smoked a pipe
John fell down
They went to the seaside
Pussy had a bath
He saw some flowers
Grannie sat on the chair
Mother sent Bill to the shop
Joan bought some ripe cherries
The children drank their milk
Fred went to the pictures
The old lady sat in the sun
The cat went to sleep on the rug
Boys like to play cricket
Many people like to swim
John ran and fell down
The baby ate his crust

Appendix III. Special Provisions in Britain for the Assessment and Educational Treatment of Deafness in Children

In the first edition of this monograph, published in 1960, there was one special Appendix on 'Audiology Clinics in Britain', and another on 'Special Schools for the Deaf and Partially Deaf'.

So rapidly did the details of these provisions change, that both of these appendices were already somewhat out of date by the time the book went into circulation.

If it is to be of any value at all, such information as was contained in these sections must be both comprehensive and up to date; but at the present time, the number of Audiology Clinics has doubled at least, and the number of Partially Hearing Units has leapt from no more than ten to the truly remarkable figure of well over a hundred.

Whilst the number and situation of special Schools for the Deaf and Partially Hearing have changed very little, the headships of some have inevitably passed into other hands, as also (in some instances) have the ages and types of children accepted by them. So too, just as inevitably, have the directorships of some of the clinics.

In any event, the important information about such schools and clinics is now readily available from other easily accessible sources. For example, the National College of Teachers of the Deaf (see Appendix IV) publishes from time to time up-to-date lists of Audiology Units and Clinics, both inside and outside the hospital services; of special Units and Schools for the Deaf and Partially Hearing, both State-controlled and privately owned; and of the names of Peripatetic Teachers of the Deaf, whether independent or attached to the various Local Educational Authorities. The most recent List of Schools is published by the British Broadcasting Corporation, 35 Marylebone High Street London WIM 4AA in a booklet entitled *I See What You Mean* (Ed: Bill Northwood) and based on a television series of the same name.

The Information Officer of the Royal National Institute for the Deaf (see Appendix V) is also able to provide, in addition to all this, regional and local lists of recognized speech therapists and instructors in lip-reading.

After very careful consideration, it has therefore been decided *not* to include these lists in this new (Third) edition, as in the second edition, but rather to give only the much more important details of those organizations which are able to keep abreast of the times.

Appendix IV. Professional Bodies Concerned with Deafness

BRITISH ASSOCIATION OF OTOLARYNGOLOGISTS
Hon. Secretary: John Ballantyne, Esq., F.R.C.S.
at the Royal College of Surgeons, 35-43, Lincoln's Inn Fields,
LONDON, WC2A 3PN
(01-405 3474)

This is a professional body of consultant ear, nose and throat specialists, and many aspects of deafness are considered by the Council and, at times and as required, by sub-committees.

The Association also has representatives on the Department of Health and Social Security's Advisory Committee on Services for Hearing Impaired People (ACSHIP).

BRITISH SOCIETY OF AUDIOLOGY
1, Birdcage Walk, LONDON, SWIH 9JJ
(01-930 7476)

CITY LITERARY INSTITUTE
(Centre for the Deaf and Speech Therapy Unit)
Keeley House, Keeley Street,
Holborn, LONDON, W.C.2.
(01-242 9872/6)

*DEPARTMENT OF AUDIOLOGY AND EDUCATION
OF THE DEAF, THE UNIVERSITY,
MANCHESTER, M13 9PL*
Director: Professor I. G. Taylor, M.D., D.P.H.
(061-273 3333)
This is the oldest unit in the British Isles for the training of Teachers of the Deaf. The course is open to qualified teachers, who can sit the examination for the Diploma of the National College of Teachers of the Deaf (q.v.) after one year's study in the department.

HEARING AND COUNCIL
226, City Road, Old Street,
LONDON, E.C.1.
(01-992 4320)

HEARING AID INDUSTRY ASSOCIATION (HAIA)
Broadway House, The Broadway,
LONDON, SW19 IRL
(01-540 3850)

LADY SPENCER-CHURCHILL COLLEGE OF EDUCATION
Wheatley, OXFORD
(0096-7 696)
There is a course here for training Teachers of Deaf Children.

THE LINK CENTRE FOR DEAFENED PEOPLE
c/o Princess Alice Memorial Hospital,
EASTBOURNE, Sussex BN21 2AX
(0323 22744)
This is a residential rehabilitation centre for those affected by sudden deafness in adult life, and for family and friends.

MEDICAL RESEARCH COUNCIL
20, Park Crescent, LONDON, W.I.
The M.R.C.'s Subcommittee on Research on Deafness has recently set up two Working Parties—one on Research Aspects of the Social and Rehabilitation Needs of the Deaf, the other on Research Aspects of the Epidemiology of Sensori-neural Hearing Loss.

At the time of writing, both working parties are nearing the end of their deliberations.

MORAY HOUSE COLLEGE OF EDUCATION
Holyrood Road, EDINBURGH, 8
(031-556 4415)

NATIONAL COLLEGE OF TEACHERS OF THE DEAF
Needwood School, Rangemore Hall,
Burton-on-Trent, STAFFORDSHIRE,
(028-371 2395)
The Diploma of The National College of Teachers of the Deaf can be taken by external students, already qualified as ordinary teachers, after a minimum of 18 months' service in a school for the deaf or partially hearing recognized by the college. A Certificate of Teacher of the Deaf is also available, to internal students of the Department of Education of the Deaf, at Manchester University.

The N.C.T.D. also publishes, from time to time, up-to-date lists of Audiology Clinics; special Schools and Units for Deaf and Partially Hearing Children; and Peripatetic Teachers of the Deaf.

SOCIETY OF AUDIOLOGY TECHNICIANS
2, Stapleton Villas,
Wordsworth Road,
LONDON, N.16

Audiology technicians are recognized as 'medical auxiliaries' by the Board of Registration of Medical Auxiliaries.

SOCIETY OF HEARING AID AUDIOLOGISTS
146, Marylebone Road,
LONDON, N.W.I.
(01-486 3638)

SOCIETY OF TEACHERS OF THE DEAF
4, Mill Green, Stoke Holy Cross,
NORWICH, NOR 55W
(050-86 2679)

This is a professional organization representing the Peripatetic Teachers of the Deaf and those in charge of Units.

UNIVERSITY OF LONDON INSTITUTE OF EDUCATION
57, Gordon Square, LONDON, W.C.1
(01-687 1500)

A department for training Teachers of the Deaf was started here in 1965.

Appendix V. Voluntary Organization for the Deaf

BREAKTHROUGH TRUST
103, Ridgeway Drive,
BROMLEY, Kent BR1 5DB
(01-857 4170)

* With the co-operation of the British Post Office, the Breakthrough Trust has recently made available equipment which enables deaf people and their relatives to communicate through the normal telephone system by means of keyboard-operated divices. Detailed information is available from: Finedon Communications Limited, 1 High Street, Finedon, Wellingborough, Northants, NN9 5JN.

BRITISH ASSOCIATION FOR THE HARD OF HEARING
(B.A.H.O.H.)
Briarfield, Syke Ings, IVER, BUCKS, SLO 9ER

BRITISH DEAF ASSOCIATION
38, Victoria Place,
CARLISLE CAI IEX
(0228 20188/9)

CHURCH OF ENGLAND COUNCIL FOR THE DEAF
Church House, Dean's Yard,
Westminster, LONDON, S.W.1.
(01-222 9011)

COMMONWEALTH SOCIETY FOR THE DEAF (C.S.D.)
75, Kinnerton Street,
LONDON, SWIX 8EU

*NATIONAL ASSOCIATION FOR DEAF-BLIND AND
RUBELLA CHILDREN*
61, Senneleys Park Road, Northfield, BIRMINGHAM, B31 OAE
(021-475 1392)

*NATIONAL COUNCIL OF WELFARE OFFICERS
TO THE DEAF* (N.C.W.O.D.)
Department of Child Care and Social Studies,
Polytechnic of North London,
62/66, Highbury Grove, LONDON, N.5
(01-359 0941)

NATIONAL DEAF-BLIND HELPERS' LEAGUE
Rainbow Court, Paston Ridings,
PETERBOROUGH, PE4 6UP
(0733 71575)

NATIONAL DEAF CHILDREN'S SOCIETY (N.D.C.S.)
General Secretary: Gordon M. L. Smith, Esq., B.A.
31, Gloucester Place, LONDON, WIH 4EA
(01-486 3251)

Founded in 1944 as the Deaf Children's Society, the N.D.C.S. became a national body in 1958.

The N.D.C.S. is concerned with the welfare and treatment (medical, surgical and educational) of deafness in children. Several booklets are produced—by otologists, educationists, parents of deaf children, and adults who were themselves born deaf. There is also an excellent quarterly magazine—*Talk*—and, since early 1958, the exhaustive and controversial 'Report on the Care of the Deaf', by J. B. Perry Robinson.

Grants have been made to assist in otological research and the training of Teachers of the Deaf, and financial assistance has been given (in special cases) to the parents of deaf children in need of commerical hearing aids.

There is a National Council, a central Committee of Management, and several sub-committees (Management, Medical Research; Education and Employment; and Finance and General Purposes) together with many regional associations.

ROYAL NATIONAL INSTITUTE FOR THE DEAF (R.N.I.D.)
105, Gower Street, LONDON, WCIE 6AH
(01-387 8033)

The R.N.I.D. was founded in 1911, as the National Bureau for promoting the General Welfare of the Deaf, and was reconstituted under the name of the National Institute for the Deaf (N.I.D.) in 1923. In 1961, on its fiftieth anniversary, it became the Royal National Institute of the Deaf (R.N.I.D.).

Apart from its welfare work, the R.N.I.D. has a large library and an active technical department, which produces (amongst other things) regular test reports on commerical hearing aids. It also provides a free testing service for hearing aids, either in London (at the new Technical Department at 321, Green Lanes, Manor House, London, N.4 (01-800 7222) or at 158, West Regent Street, Glasgow, C.2 (041-221 0794); and there is also a calibration service for audiometers. There is a number of very useful booklets covering a wide range of subjects, such as Conversation with the Deaf, Hearing Aids, and Clinical Aspects of Hearing—to name but a few.

Travelling scholarships have been awarded, from time to time, to enable those engaged in work for the deaf to visit other countries and report on their observations.

The R.N.I.D. administers eight Homes or Hostels for deaf persons, as well as one special school (Larchmoor) for maladjusted deaf children.

The Information Officer keeps up-to-date records of audiology units; hearing aid distribution centres; special schools and units for deaf and partially hearing children; peripatetic teachers of the deaf and teachers of lip-reading; further education centres for school leavers and adults; direct services provided by Local Education Authorities for deaf people; regional associations for the parents of deaf children; and clubs for the deaf and hard-of-hearing. He can also supply information about courses of training for social or welfare workers for the deaf, and about the several periodicals devoted to many different aspects of deafness.

Apart from these numerous general services, the technical department can supply a 'baby alarm', recently re-named a 'Visual Indicator'; a vibrator, mainly to waken heavy deaf sleepers; a harness, for a child's hearing aid; and a manual-alphabet version of the card game 'Kan-u-Go'.

In addition to a central Council of Management, there are several standing committees (Executive and Finance; Welfare; Publicity; Library and Information Services; Homes; Children's; and Medical and Technical.

There are also six regional associations for the deaf:

MIDLAND REGIONAL ASSOCIATION FOR THE DEAF
Birmingham Institute for the Deaf,
135, Granville Street,
BIRMINGHAM, B1 1SB
(021-643 1097)

NORTH REGIONAL ASSOCIATION FOR THE DEAF
Manchester Institute for the Deaf,
135 Grosvenor Street,
MANCHESTER, M1 7HE
(061-273 6475)

SCOTTISH REGIONAL ASSOCIATION FOR THE DEAF
Mission to the Adult Deaf and Dumb,
158 West Regent Street,
GLASGOW, G2 4RJ
(041-248 5384)

SOUTH-EAST REGIONAL ASSOCIATION FOR THE DEAF
c/o Miss C. L. Scholes, Clerk's Department,
County Hall, BEDFORD.
(0234-63222)

WELSH ASSOCIATION FOR THE DEAF
130, Windsor Road,
Penarth, GLAMORGAN CF6 1JN
(0222-25555)

WEST REGIONAL ASSOCIATION FOR THE DEAF
Institute for the Deaf,
17, St. Mary's Square,
GLOUCESTER.
(0452-20747)

The panel of four

The closing paragraph in the last edition of this monograph reads as follows: 'It is to be hoped that, in the not-too-distant future, the various organizations who work for the deaf will 'pool' their energies and resources, and it is believed that such as amalgamation would be to the enormous advantage of the deaf of all ages'.

That was in 1970, and in the following year Sir Keith Joseph, then Secretary of State for Social Security, invited the four principal organizations for the deaf to meet him for a discussion on their work and problems.

In the words of Charles Mardell (writing in *Hark*, published by the British Association of the Hard of Hearing, in the Spring of 1976): 'This invitation led to meetings of the Chairman and Secretary of the BDA, NDCS, RNID and BAHOH, to consider matters we would talk about to the Secretary of State. It was then considered a useful enterprise to make these meetings of officers a regular feature so that matters of mutual interest could be considered and united action taken. The outcome of this was the formation of the 'Panel of Four'.

Meetings with the Minister have taken place annually since 1971, the first three with Sir Keith, more recent meetings with Mr Alfred Morris, M.P., who was also responsible for setting up the Department of Health's Advisory Committee on Services for Hearing Impaired People (ACSHIP).

The Panel of Four allows the member organizations to consult one another and to take action on items which concern them all, without interfering with domestic matters or infringing upon the independence of each member. 'It has had the rewarding result', writes Mr Mardell, 'of enabling the four national bodies—(the British Deaf Association, the National Deaf Children's Society, the Royal National Institute for the Deaf and the British Association of the Hard of Hearing)—to draw closer together, to learn more about each other's work and interests and avoid duplication of effort in national subjects. Ministerial interest in the deaf and hard of hearing has never been better . . .'

BIBLIOGRAPHY

Alberti, P.W.R.M. (1964) *Journal of Laryngology and Otology*, **78**, 808.

Amman, J. C. (1692) *Surdus Loquens*, Amsterdam. English trans., by Daniel Foot, 1694, *The Talking Deaf Man*.

Ballantyne, J.C. (1951) *Journal of Laryngology and Otology*, **65**, 749.

Ballantyne, J. C. (1955) *Health Horizon*, Autumn, 49.

Ballantyne, J.C. (1957) *Talk*, Autumn, 16; Winter, 14.

Ballantyne, J. C. (1958) *Medical World* (Lond.), **89**, 118.

Ballantyne, J.C. (1959) *Proceedings of the Royal Society of Medicine*, **52**, 917.

Ballantyne, J. C. (1973) *Audiology*, **13**, 1.

Bárány, R. (1910) *Verhandlungen der Deutschenotologishe Gesellschaft*, **6**, 141.

Batten, L. W. (1957) *Proceedings of the Royal Society of Medicine*, **50**, 809.

Beales, P.H. (1957) *Journal of Laryngology and Otology*, **71**, 162.

Beales, P.H. (1957) *Journal of Laryngology and Otology*, **71**, 297.

Beales, P.H. (1958) *Journal of Laryngology and Otology*, **72**, 144.

Békésy, G. von (1947) *Acta oto-laryngologica*, **35**, 411.

Bench, R. J. (1970) *In Biomedical Engineering*, **5**, 12.

Bench, R. J. & Mentz, D. L. (1975) *Symposia of the Zoological Society of London*, **37**, 23.

Berthold, E. (1886) *Berliner Klinische Wochenschrift*, **23**, 587.

Board of Education (1938) *Report on Children with Defective Hearing*. London: H.M. Stationery Office.

Bordley, J. E., & Hardy, W. G. (1949) *Transactions of the American Otological Society*, **37**, 66

Cawthorne, T. E. (1952) In *Disease of Ear, Nose and Throat* (Ed. W. G. Scott-Brown). London: Butterworth and Co. Ltd.

Cawthorne, T.E. (1958) *Journal of Laryngology and Otology*, **72**, 281.

Dawson, M.E., Evans, M.J., Reed, M., & Minski, L. (1956) *Journal of Mental Science*, **102**, 121.

Day, K. M. (1950) *Laryngoscope*, **60**, 953.

Dickson, E. D. D. (1952) *Lancet*, **2**, 967.

Dix, M. R., Hallpike, C. S., & Hood, J. D. (1948) *Proceedings of the Royal Society of Medicine*, **41**, 516.

Douek, E.E., Gibson, W.P.R. & Humphries, K. (1973) *Journal of Laryngology and Otology*, **87**, 711.

Engström, H., Ades, H. W. & Andersson, A. (1966) *Structural Pattern of the Organ of Corti*. Stockholm: Almqvist and Wiksell.

Ewert. G. & Shea, J. J. jr (1960) *Acta oto Laryngologica*, **52**, 349.

Ewing, A. W. G. (1930) *Aphasia in Children*. London: Oxford University Press.

Ewing A. W. G. (1957) *Educational Guidance and the Deaf Child*.

Manchester: Manchester University Press.

Fisch, L. (1952) *Lancet,* **2**, 1158.

Fisch, L. (1954) *Medicine Illustrated,* **8**, 362.

Fisch, L. (1955) *Journal of Laryngology and Otology,* **69**, 479.

Fisch, L. (1955) *Lancet,* **2**, 370.

Fisch, L. (1957) *Archives of Disease in Childhood,* **32**, 230.

Fisch, L. (1957) *Journal of Laryngology and Otology,* **71**, 846.

Fisch, L. (1959) *Journal of Laryngology and Otology,* **73**, 355.

Fisch, L. (1969) *Public Health Journal of the Society of Medicine Officers of Health,* **83**, 86.

Fosbroke, J. (1830–31) *Lancet,* **1**, 533, 645, 740, 777, 823.

Fowler, E. P. (1936) *Archives of Otolaryngology,* **24**, 731.

Fowler, E.P. (1950) *Annals of Otology, Rhinology and Laryngology* (St. Louis), **59**, 980.

Fry, D. (1953) In *Diseases of Throat, Nose and Ear* (Ed. F. W. Watkyn-Thomas). London: H. K. Lewis and Co., Ltd.

Garcia-Ibanez, L. (1961) *Archives of Otolaryngology,* **73**, 268.

Gardner, L. (1957) In *The Young Handicapped Child* (Ed. A. H. Bowley). Edinburgh: E. & S. Livingstone, Ltd.

Garretson, M. D. (1969) *International Audiology,* London Congress, VIII, No. 4, p. 463.

Gesell, A. (1956) *The Volta Rewiew,* **58**, 117.

Gorman, P. (1955) *Cambridge Institute of Education Bulletin,* Summer.

Gorman, P. (1969) *Proceedings of the 4th Pan-Pacific Rehabilitation Congress,* Hong Kong.

Grime, R. P. (1975) *The Law of Noise-Induced Hearing Loss.* University of Southampton: Wolfson Unit for Noise and Vibration Control.

Hallberg, O. E. (1956) *Laryngoscope,* **66**, 1237.

Hallberg, O. E. (1957) *Journal of the American Medical Association,* **165**, 1649.

Hallpike, C.S., & Cairns, H. (1938) *Journal of Laryngology and Otology,* **53**, 625.

Hartridge, H. (1952) In *Diseases of Ear, Nose and Throat* (Ed. W. G. Scott-Brown). London: Butterworth and Co. Ltd.

Helmholtz, H. von (1863) *Tonemfindungen als physiologische Grundlage fur die Theorie der Musik,* Braunschweig. English trans. by A. E. Ellis (1885) *On the Sensations of Tone,* London.

Holmgren, G. (1922) *Acta otolaryngology,* **4**, 383.

Howarth, I. E. (1958) *Medical Officer,* **100**, 307.

Humpheries, B. (1957) *Public Health,* September.

Jackson, A. D. M. & Fisch, L. (1958) *Lancet,* **2**, 1241.

Jenkins, C. J. (1913) *Transactions of the International Congress of Medicine,* Sect. **16** (2), 609.

Jerger, J. (1960) *Journal of Speech and Hearing Disoeders,* **13**, 275.

Johnston, C. M. (1953) *British Journal of Industrial Medicine,* **10**, 41.

Kessel, J. (1876) *Archiv fur Ohrenheilkunde.,* **11**, 159.

Knight, J. J. (1967) *International Audiology*, **6**, 322.
Kodicek, J., & Garrad, J. (1955) *Journal of Laryngology and Otology*, **69**, 807.
Korkis, F. Boyes (1958) *Lancet*, **1**, 433.
Lempert, J. (1938) *Archives of Otolaryngology*, **29**, 42.
Lett, J. E. (1953) *New York Times*, January 30.
Lidén, G. (1969) *Personal Communication*.
Littler, T. S. (1954) In *Modern Trends in Diseases of Ear, Nose, and Throat* (Ed. M. Ellis) London: Butterworth and Co. Ltd.
Littler, T. S., Knight, J. J. & Strange, P. (1952) *Proceedings of the Royal Society of Medicine*, **45**, 783.
Marquet, J. F. E. (1966) *Acta otolaryngolica*, **62**, 459.
Mawson, S. (1957) *British Médical Journal*, **2**, 234.
Medical Research Council, Working Party for Research in General Practice (1957) *Lancet*, **2**, 510.
Menière, P. (1861) *Gazette medicale de Paris*, **16**, 597.
Mills, J. (1935) *A Fugue—tn Cycles and Bels*. London: Chapman and Hall.
Ministry of Education, Pamphlet No. 30 (1956) *Education of the Handicapped Pupil*. London: H.M. Stationery Office.
Ministry of Education, List 42 (1956) *List of Special Schools for Handicapped Pupils in England and Wales*. London: H.M. Stationery Office.
Ministry of Health (1957) *Memorandum on the Prevention and Alleviation of Deafness*.
Montgomery, G. W. G. (1966) *American Annals of the Deaf*, **111**, 557.
Morgans, M. E. & Trotter, W. R. (1958) *Lancet*, **1**, 607.
Morrison, A. W. (1957) *Management of Sensorineural Deafness*, London: Butterworths.
Moulonguet, A., & Bouche,J.(1952) *Annals of Otolaryngology*, **69**, 71.
Northwood, B. (1975) *I see what you mean* (B.B.C. Publications), Editor.
Ormerod, F.C., & Mc Lay, K. (1956) *Journal of Laryngology and Otology*, **70**, 648.
Ormerod. F.C. (1957) *Journal of Laryngology and Otology*, **71**, 427.
Passe, E. R. Garnett (1951) *Lancet*, **1**, 783.
Passe, E. R. Garnett (1953) *Archives of Otolaryngology*, **3**, 257.
Passow, K. (1899) *Verhandlungen deutsch otolaryngologische*, **6**, 141.
Portmann, M., & Claverie, G. (1957) *Annals of Otology Rhinology and Laryngology* (St. Louis), **66**, 49.
Proctor, C. A., & Proctor, B. (1967) *Archives of Otolaryngology*, **85**, 23.
Quigley, S. P. (1969) *The Influence of Finger-spelling on the Development of Language, Communication and Educational Achievements of Deaf Children*. Institute for Research into Exceptional Children: University of Illinois.

Quigley, S. (1969) *International Audiology*, London Congress, VIII, No. 4, p. 472.

Rainer, J. D. & Altshuler, K. Z. (1969) *International Audiology, London Congress*, VIII, No. 4. p. 435.

Rawson, Annette (1973) *Deafness: Report of a Departmental Enquiry into the Promotion of Research*, London: H.M.S.O.

Reed, M. (1956) *Talk*, Winter, 14.

Robinson, J. B. Perry (1958) *Report for the National Deaf Children's Society on the Care of the Deaf*. London: National Deaf Children's Society.

Rosen, S. (1952) *Archives of Otolaryngology*, **56**, 610.

Rosen, S. (1953) *New York State Journal of Medicine*, **53**, 2650.

Rosen, S., & Bergman, M. (1954) *Acta otolaryngologica, Suppl.* **118**, 180.

Rosen, S. (1955) *Acta otolaryngologica*, **45**, 532.

Rosen, S. (1956) *Archives of otolaryngology*, **64**, 227.

Rosen, S. (1958) *Journal of Laryngology and Otology*, **72**, 263.

Scottish Council for Research in Education (1956) *Hearing Defects in Schoolchildren*. London: University of London Press.

Sheridan, M. D. (1944) *British Medical Journal*, **2**, 272.

Sheridan, M. D. (1945) *British Medical Journal*, **1**, 707.

Sheridan, M. D. (1955) *Medical World* (London), **82**, 146.

Sheridan, M. D. (1958) *British Medical Journal*, **2**, 999.

Sheridan, M. D. (1959) *Proceedings of the Royal Society of Medicine*, **52**, 913.

Sourdille, M. (1929) *Bulletin de l'Academie de Médiecin*, **102**, 674.

Stevenson, R. Scott, & Guthrie, D. (1949) *A History of Otolaryngology*. Edinburgh: E. & S. Livingstone, Ltd.

Stevenson, R. Scott (1951) *In A Harley Street Mirror*. London: Christopher Johnson.

Stevenson, R. Scott (1954) *Goodbye, Harley Street*. London: Christopher Johnson.

Stevenson, R. Scott (1954) In *Modern Trends in Diseases of the Ear, Nose and Throat* (Ed. M. Ellis). London: Butterworth & Co., Ltd.

Terkildsen, K., & Thomsen, K.A. (1959) *Journal of Laryngology and Otology*.

Thouless, R. H. (1957) *Report of the Conference of Audiology Workers*, Cambridge, July 21.

Waardenburg, P.J. (1951) *American Journal of Human Genetics*, **3**, 195.

Watkyn-Thomas, F. W. (1952) In *Diseases of Throat, Nose and Ear* (Ed. F. W. Watkyn-Thomas). London: H. K. Lewis & Co., Ltd.

Wever, E. G., & Bray, P. W., (1930) *Proceedings of the National Academy of Sciences of the United States of America*, **16**, 344.

Wever, E. G. (1949) *Theory of Hearing*. New York: John Wiley.

Wright, D. (1969) *Deafness: A Personal Account*. Allen Lane, The Penguin Press.

Wullstein, H. (1953) *Proceedings of the Fifth International Congress of Oto-Rhino-Laryngology* Amsterdam: Excepta Medica Foundation, p. 104.

Zöllner, E. (1955) *Journal of Laryngology and Otology,* **69**, 637.

Index